Praise for *Give Back the Light*

"Retina surgeons are the crème de la crème in the realm of ophthalmology. Steve Charles stands right at the top of that pyramid. Moore does a masterful job of combining his compelling personal struggle as a patient with clear explanations of eye structures, ophthalmic procedures, and the innovative techniques and instruments that Dr. Charles has developed to preserve our precious vision. As someone who has covered the momentous achievements of the retina community for almost two decades, it is a joy to see the accomplishments of this wondrous eye surgeon finally celebrated."

—**Jerry Helzner,** News Editor, *Retinal Physician Magazine*

"James Moore sneaks a comprehensive education into an intimate and inspiring true story of one man's greatest passion intersecting with another man's greatest fear. A poignant and compelling journey of discovery about the mysteries of human vision, technology, and the relentlessness of hope."

—**Kristen Tsetsi,** author, *The Age of the Child*

"James Moore has written a truly original book about hope and discovery—the story of one man's search to save his sight and a remarkable doctor whose gift for invention and skills as a surgeon have helped restore vision to millions. The author writes about astonishing medical procedures with clarity and precision, deeply reported and rich in detail. And he uncovers the little-known history of medical giants in pursuit of the impossible. This is a profound book, both poignant and exhilarating, and readers will come away with the knowledge that Moore has taken them somewhere totally new."

—**Wayne Slater,** Writer Emeritus, *Dallas Morning News*

"*Give Back the Light* is a tremendous achievement. James C. Moore weaves a wrenching personal account of his struggle to save the sight in his right eye with the history and accomplishments of legendary eye surgeon and innovator, Dr. Steve Charles. The book combines brilliant storytelling and a testament to one of the great minds in eye surgery with questions about where the divide lies between patient and physician responsibility. This book is a mesmerizing dive into the recent history of eye surgery and the journey of one patient."

—**Mary Pauline Lowry,** author, *Wildfire*

"This remarkable book combines Jim Moore's battle to keep the vision in his right eye with a highly readable explanation of the history and intricacies of eye surgery (proliferative vitreo retinopathy, anyone?). It's a profile of a modern medical hero: Dr. Steve Charles, who also happens to be an engineer, an ace inventor, and a jet-airplane pilot. It's easy to be cynical about today's world. This is a book about an inspirational doctor who has saved the eyesight of thousands of people. It will open your eyes to the beauty, the miracle of seeing."

—**Robert Bryce,** author, *Smaller Faster Lighter Denser Cheaper: How Innovation Keeps Proving the Catastrophists Wrong*

GIVE BACK THE LIGHT

Also by James Moore

Bush's Brain: How Karl Rove Made George W. Bush Presidential

Bush's War for Reelection: Iraq, the White House, and the People

The Architect: Karl Rove and the Master Plan for Absolute Power

In the Time of Man, Science Fiction

The Rembrandt Bomb, with Chuck Klinger, Fiction, Thriller

Adios Mofo: Why Rick Perry Will Make America Miss George W. Bush

GIVE BACK THE LIGHT

A Doctor's Relentless Struggle to End Blindness

JAMES C. MOORE

New York Times BEST-SELLING AUTHOR

WITH STEVE CHARLES, M.D.

GREENLEAF
BOOK GROUP PRESS

The names and identifying characteristics of persons referenced in this book have been changed to protect their privacy.

Published by Greenleaf Book Group Press
Austin, Texas
www.gbgpress.com

Distributed by Greenleaf Book Group

For ordering information or special discounts for bulk purchases, please contact Greenleaf Book Group at PO Box 91869, Austin, TX 78709, 512.891.6100.

Design and composition by Greenleaf Book Group and Kim Lance
Cover design by Greenleaf Book Group and Kim Lance

Publisher's Cataloging-in-Publication data is available.

Print ISBN: 978-1-62634-562-1

eBook ISBN: 978-1-62634-563-8

Part of the Tree Neutral® program, which offsets the number of trees consumed in the production and printing of this book by taking proactive steps, such as planting trees in direct proportion to the number of trees used: www.treeneutral.com

Printed in the United States of America on acid-free paper

18 19 20 21 22 23 10 9 8 7 6 5 4 3 2 1

First Edition

To my father,

James Clinton Moore

And all the things that might have been

"Ring the bells that still can ring.
Forget your perfect offering.
There is a crack, a crack in everything.
That's how the light gets in."

LEONARD COHEN,
"ANTHEM"

Contents

Foreword

BY CHRISTOPHER F. BLODI, M.D.

Attempting to capture the essence of Steve Charles is a daunting task for any author, yet James Moore has done just that. Moore has interwoven his own catastrophic retinal detachment with the life story of the retinal surgeon, Dr. Charles. Sadly, by the time Charles examined Moore, the detachment was inoperable. That end result provides several lessons for the reader: the harrowing experience of a patient losing eyesight in spite of repeated procedures, the life forces that have molded Charles into a near-mythical eye surgeon, and a better understanding of the way that exceptional individuals, in any field, work and perform.

This book will appeal to three types of readers. First, those interested in their own medical problems will be able to learn from the ways that the author confronted the health care system and the ways needed to deal with medical failure and adjust to a new disability. Second, the book will be useful to those that enjoy learning about the very driven people in modern society with a need to always push their field of work forward. Reading the life story of a Steve Jobs and his role bringing the computer to the home, or of a Dian Fossey and her obsession with understanding and protecting the Silverback gorillas of central Africa, can let the reader begin to understand how and why some of us are able to contribute so much to society. Finally, ophthalmologists, and retinal surgeons in particular, will enjoy learning more about Dr. Charles, someone who has dominated his field of retinal surgery for almost fifty years.

I have known Steve Charles for thirty-five years. During conversations held in locations ranging from Nantucket Island to Hawaii to his home in Memphis, I have learned that the real Steve Charles is extraordinarily similar to the public Steve Charles. The rapid-fire speech pattern is always there—as if to say that time is short and many ideas need to be presented. The compelling desire to forcefully take a stand on a controversial medical issue (such as a surgical strategy) exists for day-to-day matters, as well. Charles has never been afraid to say exactly where he stands on any issue, from surgical techniques to religious views.

Through the years, Charles has steadily advanced his chosen field of retinal surgery. He has developed almost innumerable surgical techniques and instruments. The family influences are strong. One grandfather was a surgeon, the other an engineer. His father was an artist whose academic career centered on sculpting. All were different and important role models for Charles.

Sometimes, fate and fortuitous timing are important in one's career path. Certainly, this was the case with Charles. Growing up in Miami, it was only natural for him to enroll there in medical school (after undergraduate training in engineering). And it was his good fortune to continue his training to be an eye surgeon at the University of Miami's Bascom Palmer Eye Institute. It was here that he met and trained with such pioneering retinal surgeons as David Kasner, who first popularized the very idea of vitreous surgery, and Robert Machemer, who refined the technique. All of this pushed Charles further forward.

However, not all influences are external. Charles' extremely driven personality comes from within. This is a man with almost no hobbies, a man able to perform ten microsurgical retinal operations per day, at age 75, without any skill degradation whatsoever. Charles continues, relentlessly, to care for patients, develop new surgical equipment, and travel the world to provide charity care and teach others. His mind-set remains that physicians should always learn and change their techniques for the better. He serves as a model for all private practice health care providers by taking on all patients that need him, from children of indigent families living in the Mississippi Delta to Elvis Presley, regardless of a patient's financial circumstances.

Virtually all that Charles does is for a specific and exact reason. This is true for everything from how he runs his medical practice to how he keeps himself fit. I once talked to him about his unusual and well-known lecture technique. A Steve Charles lecture is always delivered with a mile-a-minute speech rate and almost innumerable PowerPoint slides that are chock-full of statistical details and seemingly too much information.

"Why this brutal style of speaking?" I asked him.

"Well, I do it on purpose," he said. "I just want to get out as much information as possible in the time that's been allotted for me to use. I figure that anyone with questions can come and talk to me after I'm finished."

James Moore, by writing about his own misfortune, has given us valuable insight into the ways of this driven individual. Moore's background as a writer and commentator have helped produce an enjoyable and smoothly-written story. The lay reader will learn more about the toll an illness can take on a person and how one can persevere through the challenge. The ophthalmologist will learn more about Steve Charles (hopefully not feeling, as I often do, as a mere epigone). All readers will appreciate the single-mindedness that allows some humans to positively impact at least one small part of modern life.

Christopher F. Blodi, M.D.
Des Moines, Iowa
June 2018

Preface

There are books an author wants to write and few that they must write. I was unable to avoid the topics addressed in this narrative. There was also a matter of counterintuitive conflict; the central character in this story is inspirational while the circumstances for me, the narrator, were quite depressing. I felt this contradiction offered intrigue. This is best explained more specifically by saying that while I was struggling to save the vision in my right eye, I came across one of the most amazing people I had ever encountered in more than four decades of journalism, travel, and curiosity.

A book demanded itself.

My part of the story is troubling and not just on a personal level. As a robustly healthy man, I did not have much experience with doctors and hospitals and surgeons. Generally, I went to see my physician every now and again for a checkup and was told to go enjoy my life, which I did with great relish. When my retina tore, though, and then detached, I entered into a health care system that demanded a very high level of vigilance, which was almost impossible to exercise. Even with an education and a level of experience outside of most people, I discovered I was not prepared for the nuances that made the difference between excellence and average care.

The greater problem, in my view, is not the cost of health care in the U.S. but the varying ranges of competence on the part of doctors. How can a patient expect to know what they are getting? After each failed surgery to save my vision, I began to wonder about my doctor's skills and training. Retinal reattachment, while not quite mundane, was performed with great success every day around the world. Why did my retina consistently fail to stay attached post-operatively? The options were only that I bore a physiology in my eye that was sufficiently peculiar that the oils, laser, and gas were unable to sustain a pressure and contact that led to healing, or my surgeon lacked a competence that was up to the task of my biology. My sense after my experience was that much of my problem had to do with a doctor whose level of skill was good enough for routine retinal procedures but made more complicated operations higher risk than they might have been in the hands of someone with more experience and talent. A second opinion from an accomplished retinal surgeon, however, suggested every procedure had been performed with care and competence.

If a doctor treats mostly basic cases, and does not attend seminars and conferences to learn the latest surgical techniques of his or her specialty, how is that individual ever going to be prepared when the outlier comes into their office? The biology of the human eye is the same in everyone, but some have thinner retinas; the globe of the eye is longer or shorter; we might heal faster than someone else; the back of an eye is decidedly more curved in a near-sighted person, and the retina might be more likely to detach because there is not a flatness that is present in a correctly proportioned eye. All of these dynamics make each retinal surgery more than a simple procedure, yet most patients recover and have fine eyesight.

A modern doctor's obligation, though, in the world's most technologically advanced and wealthiest culture is not just to the simple cases. A vitreoretinal surgeon needs to be capable of repairing the most profoundly damaged of eyes, and, much like an airline pilot, also train for moments they are likely to never experience. I do not believe my retinal surgeon was incompetent; I think he was average and capable, and my eye was a profound challenge to him, which he seemingly never acknowledged because he thought standard practices would correct my issue. Regardless of his Ivy League education, university internships and fellowships, and training in trauma rooms of a major metropolitan hospital, he was not up to the task, nor, do I suppose, was I equal to the challenge of being well enough informed to ask the right questions.

But is that a patient's job? Are we supposed to be educated about medicine when seeking care or must we trust the education and training of our surgeons? In the course of the almost five years I struggled with my eye, I became well-educated about the eye, and, most especially, the retina. I might have asked better questions had I been as informed when I went in for my initial pars plana vitrectomy to remove the vitreous from my eye and reattach my retina. I was not without information, though, and was consistently bothered by the contradicting answers provided by my surgeon. Ultimately, I concluded I was a victim of his limited abilities.

Which constantly prompts a question from friends: Why didn't you sue?

The answer is relatively easy for me. I do not see how a man who has passed his boards to be qualified at the peak of his profession can be considered incompetent. He was, and is, talented enough to help a lot of people. In fact, he has opened a clinic that provides care to the indigent with eye problems. I simply happened to be a statistical outlier that was beyond his ken. A lawsuit might have harmed his practice, ruined his ability to help others, and it would have only brought me a minor settlement from his insurance company, which would have raised his rates. Further, I would have been unable to get on with my life and work. There seemed to be no value in hurting a man for being good at his job 98 percent of the time.

There was more pragmatism than altruism in my decision. I wanted to get back to my regular routines of work and travel after years of surgery, and even after constant research, I realized there were no discernible standards for surgical repair results after a retinal tear and detachment. Every case, obviously, was unique. The Texas legal system would also offer little hope of satisfaction either. Tort reform laws capped penalties in medical malpractice cases and damages for loss of work might never be awarded by skeptical juries. I was probably not going to be satisfied with a legal outcome, and it would only be more years of worrying as lawyers waited for an insurance company settlement that was likely to do little more than cover their time and expenses.

Before I had even worked through that calculus, though, I became determined to find the best possible retinal surgeon practicing in America and see if I might gain access. The search led me, improbably, to Memphis, and the Charles Retina Institute. Steve Charles, I had discovered, had performed more retinal surgeries than anyone in history and developed many of the technologies and operational techniques used to save vision and reattach retinas. His list of achievements, I discovered, was improbable, and the more I learned about Dr. Charles, the more determined I became to tell his story.

In fact, I found it patently absurd that Steve Charles was hardly known outside of his profession. His work, arguably, has saved the eyesight of millions of people around the world through the advancement of his surgical platforms, tools, and various procedures he perfected to save the retina. He spoke from podiums at conferences all over the globe, did demonstration and educational surgeries, and seemingly had time for everyone who approached him. The doctor had also raised three daughters, an entrepreneur and two physicians, and flew his own twin-engine jet. His work ethic of seeing dozens of patients on Monday and Wednesday, operating on Tuesday and Thursday, and then traveling to teach and consult on weekends, is mind-boggling for even the most energetic of observers, and at age 75, the doctor shows no traces of decline.

Mostly, though, I felt fortunate to be able to tell this man's story. Steve is humble but aware of his personal exceptionalism. Regardless, he expects nothing of others that he does not demand of himself, which is why, undoubtedly, he has built such a dedicated and loyal staff in Memphis. My only concern about this project is that I would not be able to do justice to Steve Charles, M.D., and the people whose lives he has impacted with his research and surgery. I would consider that a fine personal accomplishment in my life of writing and reporting, and I have made a great effort to learn engineering, biology, and medicine, to make certain I am able to comprehend the breadth of Charles' mind and his work.

And I hope this book does justice to his great legacy.

ONE

Some Sad Things Known to Man

Memphis did not seem like the city where I might solve a complex medical problem. Nothing, though, was making sense to me at this point in my struggle to save the sight in my right eye. I had recently passed my driver's license vision exam with one eye and was rolling up the Natchez Trace in Mississippi, taking a scenic run to Memphis with my daughter in the hope that I might be able to distract myself from the curtain of darkness that had fallen over the right side of my face. The Ross Barnett Reservoir glistened in the spring afternoon, and the reflected sunlight broke into diamonds and made me smile. I was becoming melancholy about the beauty of the world and what, if anything, I might miss if I ended up with only one good eye.

My Austin retina surgeon, Dr. D, had mentioned the name of a physician in Memphis who was considered without peer in his microsurgical subspecialty, and I had sought him out online. Though I had spent more than three decades as a journalist and was not easily intimidated, as I read the CV of Dr. Steve Charles on his website,

I wondered if I had any chance of getting his care. He was a physician and design engineer and had generated market-leading sales for companies that had developed, manufactured, and sold his surgical systems; his ingenuity had led to various critical techniques used in retinal operations. He had performed an estimated 38,000 vitreoretinal surgeries, more than anyone in history.

There was a contact form on the site, which I filled out and submitted. I assumed that I might hear from a clerical assistant in a week or so on my remote chances of getting in to see Dr. Charles within a few months. Instead, in less than five minutes, in the dead of night, I had a personal email from the doctor himself.

I had written, "I have had multiple surgeries to repair my retina. It started out with a tear that became a detachment, and none of the surgical efforts of my doctor to reattach it have been successful. I have been facedown with gas for many weeks, several times, and have endured silicone oil and multiple laser surgeries. I don't know what to do. Can you offer me any advice?"

"Yes, please come see me in Memphis," he wrote. "I am sorry this has happened to you. I am copying my assistant, and she will put you on a VIP list so you can get a quick appointment."

"Really? I'm not any kind of a VIP, Dr. Charles. But I'd sure like to have you look at my eye."

"You are a VIP to me because you need care and need it fast. Let's get you to Memphis as soon as possible."

My expectations were not high when my daughter and I walked into the Charles Retina Institute only a few days later. I had researched problems with the retina and the use of lasers and oils and gas, and I was fairly confident that my options had been exhausted. I did not know much about Charles beyond the fact that my surgeon had told me he was the best available, probably in the world. I had learned a bit more about him from his website. Now, I was sitting in a somewhat darkened room with my eye dilated, anticipating my exam. The fact that my pupil could still be dilated and my iris continued to look relatively colorful and liquid gave me some hope that my eye's health remained viable.

"Do you think he can fix it, Daddy?" my daughter, Amanda Noelle, in her mid-20s, had asked. She had never known me to experience a health problem beyond sniffles or an upset stomach, and she had never seen me in the grip of any personal fear.

"I don't know, baby. If anyone can, I think he is the guy."

I was summoned for a series of photos that attempted to capture the state of my retina, then taken down a long hallway into an examining room and invited to sit. I could hear the doctor's voice down a hall that ran parallel to the corridor I had just traversed. I assumed he moved from exam to exam along this private passageway. As his voice came closer, I tried to brighten my grim perspective.

"This is the gentleman who came up from Texas," said his assistant, Sabrina Newsom.

"Oh, yes, my online friend. The author. Well, let's have a look."

Steve Charles was unimposing, a bit over six feet tall with an athletic presence, but his unmistakable confidence filled the room. He used his thumb to press my upper eyelid against my brow and then swung his light over my eye to examine the retina. He could get no view to the retina because of blood in the eye, and he subsequently used an ultrasound to get an accurate image. My doctor back in Austin, unable to effectively use ultrasound to see my retina, had been struggling for several weeks to give me a long-term prognosis.

I had resolved to see Dr. Charles after I reached an emotional low point: On my way to one of my last appointments with Dr. D. I was so distraught that I pulled into an empty parking lot and cried while sitting in my truck, a grown, gray-haired man lost in personal grief among an expanse of outlet stores. Laughter would have been a more logical response in that setting. After I regained my composure, I called my friend Greg in Houston. We had been as close as brothers for decades, and he instinctively understood my fear for my eye.

"Nothing's working," I said.

"I thought everything worked these days. Laser and whatever else they do. Retina detachments are treatable, aren't they?"

"Yeah, they are, but . . ."

"But what?"

"I don't know. Maybe I've just got bum genetics. Or even a bad doctor. He seems competent, but contradictions turn up in his prognoses, and he isn't really consistent in what he tells me."

"Well, you need to figure that out, buddy. You can't have someone incompetent messing with your eyesight."

Greg was right, of course. I had been worrying about these same issues for almost four years, since I had discovered a problem with my retina. Sitting in front of the television one afternoon, I had noticed dark flecks floating through my field of vision. They appeared almost like insects, but floaters had long bothered me, and I did not think I was experiencing a potentially serious issue with my eyesight. Perhaps, I thought, a few more floaters had accumulated as I had aged.

My optometrist worked me into his appointment schedule the next day and ran a color scan of my retina. The machine he used was a non-mydriatic retinal fundus camera. That meant it provided detailed color images of the retina, the thin tissue that lines the back hemisphere of the eye and captures light for the optic nerve to process as moving images for the human brain. Non-mydriatic technology does not call for dilation of the pupils, normally required to expand the field of vision for ophthalmologists examining the retina and the interior of the eye.

"Hmmmm . . ." said the young technician, who was recording the images as I tried to keep my eyelids open.

"What are you *hmming* about?" I asked.

"Oh, nothing, I'm sure. We'll get this to the doctor right away."

There *was* something, however, and as I waited for the optometrist, I wondered what the assistant might have discovered. My vision had never been good. From the time I was four years old I had worn what the other kids had referred to as "Coke-bottle glasses" with thick lenses to correct my nearsightedness. The shape of my eye was longer than optimal, and my point of focus was in front of the macula, the highly pigmented oval near the center of the retina, which is responsible for delivering the sharpest vision to the eye. I saw almost nothing with clarity that was more than a few feet distant.

"I think it looks like there is a retinal tear on this image."

The optometrist, a family friend who had built a busy practice, did not appear overly concerned as he stared at the computer. He pointed at a spot on the confusingly colorful screen where blood veins and shadows made comprehension almost impossible for the nonmedical observer.

"I guess I don't see it," I said.

"It's right here."

He laid his finger against a dark line that emerged against the whitish background. "I'm quite certain this is a retinal tear."

"Which means what?"

"You need to get to a specialist."

A retinal tear leading to a detachment of the retina would be problematic, and even debilitating, to personal health and employment if it were to go untreated. I knew little more than the high school biology basics of the human eye. I understood the functions of the pupil and cornea, the properties of the retina, and how rods and cones worked to distinguish the light and colors delivered to the optic nerve. But I had never heard of vitreous, the fibrous, clear gel that fills the interior of the eye. Vitreous is partially composed of millions of tiny collagen fibers that are attached to the delicate retina, and if there is a tear or a hole in the retina, fluid can leak under the retina and cause a detachment, leading to loss of vision. Or the vitreous can pull on the retina and create the same problem.

The optometrist gave me a card for a retinal specialist who had recently opened an office in North Austin. When I called the next morning and described my diagnosis, he said I should come to his office immediately and they would work me into his schedule. Although there was a sense of urgency in his voice, I did not quite understand the apparent concern. My eyesight was unchanged, and the previous floaters were no longer visible. In fact, I debated whether I should even bother keeping the appointment.

My health had always been robust, and injuries like cuts and broken bones had healed fast enough that doctors often were amazed. Once in my early 50s, after snapping both bones of my forearm while playing baseball and undergoing surgery to insert a plate, I was back playing catch and lightly swinging a bat less than three weeks later. Was it not possible that my eye might also heal and the retina reattach naturally along the line of the tear?

Philosophically, I have always chosen to avoid doctors, medication, and any type of invasive procedure, if possible. I'm not averse to doctors, though, and do not hesitate to run to their care when it's needed. Consequently, I saw no harm in having this specialist conduct an examination.

After my eye was dilated, Dr. D peered through the pupil to assess the health of the retina. His conclusion seemed a bit abrupt.

"We are going to have to put in some laser," he said.

"Okay, what does that mean?"

I ask doctors questions. Hell, I pester almost everyone for information, from strangers in airport bars to those I meet on the running trail. When it came to my eye, I needed to know almost as much as the retinal specialist. Nothing was going to be done to it until I understood the risks.

"You have a small tear. We will use the laser, here in the office, and put in laser spots around the tear. The light does a slight burn on the retina, and as it heals, it reattaches to the layer under the retina. The vitreous stops flowing through the tear and detaching the retina."

"Is this serious?"

"No, it shouldn't be. Most tears can be repaired with laser, and the patient's vision is never impaired."

"Okay, we can do this now?"

"Yes, certainly."

As I leaned back in the exam chair, I saw the doctor's degrees and training certifications framed on the wall. An Ivy Leaguer with about 20 years of medical training and residencies at university and municipal hospitals, Dr. D came across as low key but knowledgeable. It seemed natural for me to trust his skills and experience.

Unfortunately, almost four years later, I was sitting in an exam chair at Charles Retina Institute in Memphis, hoping for a miracle. There was no way for me to know if my monocular blindness was a consequence of surgical incompetence or just the genetics of a long eye, since the longer the eyeball's shape, the harder it becomes for the retina to be flattened against the back after tears, holes, and detachments. Over time, Dr. D had tried a series of procedures that involved the removal of the vitreous, laser treatments, replacing the vitreous with silicone oil, and using gas bubbles. Not one had succeeded in fixing my right eye.

As Dr. Charles was conducting his examination that morning, he made a statement that I found astounding—and devastating.

"This shouldn't have happened to you. And if you'd been in my care, it probably would not have happened to you."

Whether opinion or simple fact, the assertion was almost impossible for me to process. I began to think I was a victim of incompetence and a medical system that demands too much of the patient. How is anyone supposed to know a surgeon's capabilities without hours of extensive research? Eventually, I would come to understand why Steve Charles was so assured and capable and what he knew that another retinal surgeon, even one Ivy League trained, did not. My immediate question, however, was whether he might still be able to give me back my sight.

When I had initially begun my research on his achievements, Dr. Charles struck me as an unknown yet historical figure. Probably no one person had a broader impact on vision and ophthalmological surgery than this doctor. His inventions of machines, tools, and new techniques were transformative for retinal surgery, and they have improved outcomes for thousands of people wanting desperately to see. And yet almost no one outside of his professional field knew who he was or what he had accomplished. I would come to know much more about Steve Charles. But I was already growing convinced that if anyone could give me back my eyesight, it would be this doctor.

And I just wanted to see.

TWO

Giants in the Room

A uniquely American institution, Bascom Palmer Eye Institute (BPEI) in Miami has had a sweeping and profound impact on the advancement of eye care, and, in fact, gets credit for developing the critical vitrectomy procedure to repair most damaged retinas. Until doctors and an engineer at BPEI had designed the technology and the procedures for removing vitreous from the interior of the eye, most surgical interventions for the retina were arguably guesswork that used everything from needles to heat and even a type of rubber band. The arrival in Miami of a doctor from Germany after World War II, followed by an engineer from Australia, led to a revolution in how surgery was performed on the interior of the human eye. Steve Charles would be at BPEI to witness and participate in the dawning of these advancements.

The beginning of that story was recorded with a black-and-white photo. Even in the hottest Miami summers, Robert Machemer, M.D., was never seen without his lab coat while performing research or eye surgery. This day, in the humid, stifling garage at his home, where his work and image were about to be rendered onto film, was no exception.

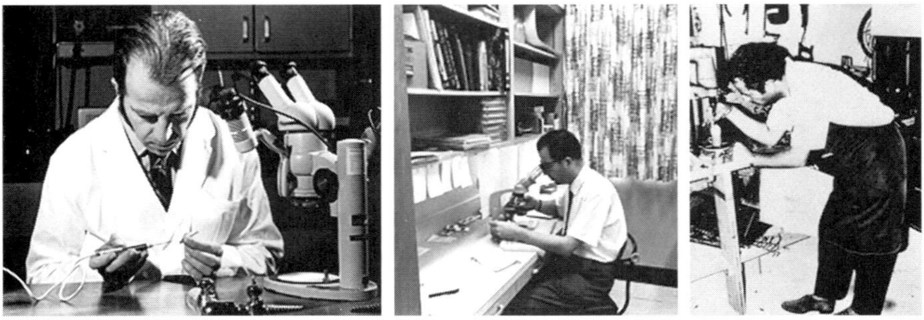

Dr. Robert Machemer, M.D. (Courtesy of Bascom Palmer Eye Institute)

The serious and bespectacled son of a Nazi battlefield surgeon, Machemer had thick, dark hair and long sideburns that suggested he might have been anything other than a doctor. In fact, he was on the verge of dramatically altering techniques for operating on the eye. The procedure was to become known as pars plana vitrectomy (PPV), the removal of the vitreous substance from the inner chamber of the eye by insertion of an instrument through the front, near the cornea. Vitreous is the clear, gelatinous material filled with fine collagen fibers that attach to the retina, the delicate light-gathering tissue that lines the scleral wall, generally behind the equator of the eye. Light passes through the vitreous and is perceived by the retinal tissue. Historically, doctors had limited success repairing detached or torn retinas because of complications caused by the presence of vitreous; it tended to stretch and pull at the delicate tissue, causing complications and damage. Machemer became convinced the clear substance was not critical to the eye's function, and he had a plan and a tool for the removal of vitreous.

Which is why he was standing over an upright egg with a drill in hand.

The photo really wasn't meant to be serious, according to Jean-Marie Parel, a Ph.D. physicist, who engineered another instrument that Machemer eventually used to enter the eye. "We just wanted to show you could drill inside of something delicate like an egg," said Parel in an interview years later. "When you turned the drill, it literally sucked stuff up out of the egg. Robert wanted to prove you could use the drill as a flute, and the egg yolk and white matter would come up. This was his way of showing we could do it ourselves—remove the vitreous from the eye in a safe and fairly nonintrusive way."

Parel had ended up in Miami after leaving his home in France and working at the University of Melbourne in Australia. He and Machemer had been recruited to join BPEI, a new research and treatment facility at the University of Miami, founded by Edward W.D. Norton, M.D., a stout Irishman with a gentle voice and a facility for identifying doctors with drive, skill, and scientific curiosity.

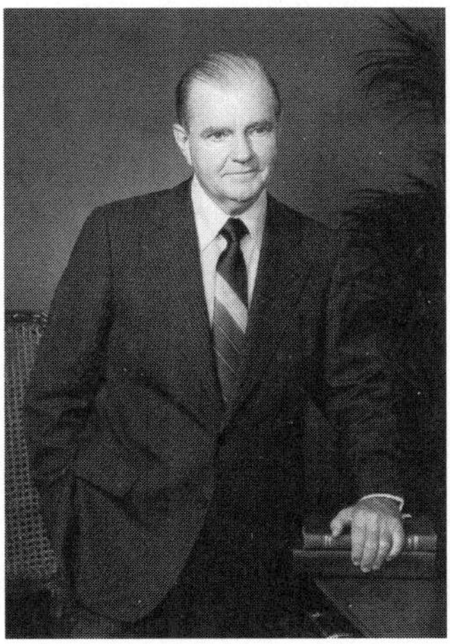

Edward W. D. Norton, founder, Bascom Palmer Eye Institute

Parel, slender, intense, and brimming with ideas, had met Norton at an international conference and had shown the Miami physician drawings he had made of a device to cut up vitreous. Unfortunately,

Parel had not included a methodology for extracting vitreous from the eye. But his ingenious thinking had almost immediately convinced the visionary Norton that he needed to hire Parel.

Norton was wasting no time in trying to build a center of excellence for eye surgery and research. Only three years after being named the medical school's chief of the Department of Ophthalmology in 1958, he had managed to generate enough money to break ground on the BPEI building. Norton soon began to develop his faculty and staff with some of the brightest young minds in medicine. They included Dave Sime, M.D., a brilliant cataract surgeon who happened to be a former Olympic medalist and future grandfather of a Heisman Trophy candidate and National Football League player. Dr. David Kasner, a New York City transplant, was nearby, teaching residents at the Veterans' Administration hospital and serving as an unpaid member of BPEI's clinical faculty. Kasner had become an ophthalmologist after being deeply affected by his brother's loss of sight in one eye. He is credited with developing the first historical technique for removing vitreous, which is what had attracted the attention of Machemer.

BPEI's medical advancements paralleled NASA's development, and although he might never have thought of the comparison, Ed Norton's institution was a similar gathering of inquisitive and analytical minds that was also to have an impact on the human condition. His institute made numerous changes that transformed ophthalmology, especially of the retina, cataract surgery using intraocular lenses, and the design and creation of microsurgical instruments and procedures. Many of those would be offered eventually by the young Steve Charles, who had studied mechanical and electrical engineering and pre-med at North Carolina State and the University of Oklahoma and had practically talked his way into medical school at Miami.

"When I was interviewed before admission," Charles recalled, "I was asked what I could bring to the medical school that others couldn't. I said, 'Instrumentation. You want things hooked up, don't you? And have electronics that need to be built or kept running? I can do that.' I ended up being at Bascom Palmer at an amazing time. I was just so fortunate, and I am still incredibly grateful for my experiences there."

Charles had completed four of the five years needed to graduate from the engineering program at the University of Oklahoma when he was distracted by a program combining engineering with pre-med. Bringing together the disciplines of engineering and medicine was logical and maybe even a bit familial to Charles. His father's oldest brother, John David Charles, Steve's godfather, had been a leading colorectal surgeon, and his grandfather, Clayton Henry Charles, had spent his medical career doing emergency operations on lumberjacks in the woods of Wisconsin before moving to Milwaukee and specializing in surgery.

Steve Charles' mechanical aptitude likely came from his maternal grandfather, Harry Godfrey Johnson, a Swedish immigrant, who designed diesel engines after working for years in the Elgin Watch factory. The creative penchant for designing and building systems and devices, though, seems to have descended from his father, Clayton, who was known widely as a sculptor, painter, city planner, and art historian. Clayton had studied with the famed sculptor Henry Moore, had a master's in art history from the University of Wisconsin, and had been a professor at several universities before concluding his career as chairman of the Art Department at the University of Miami. Charles' mother, Madeline, had also studied art history.

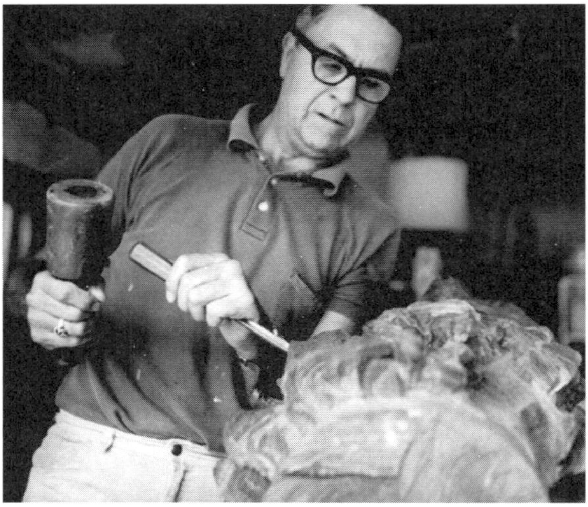

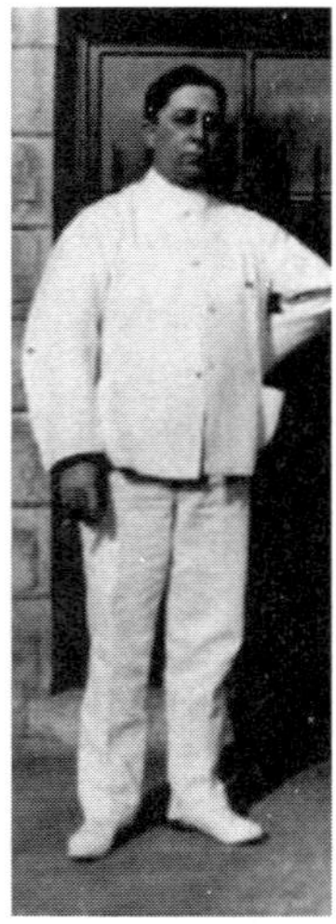

(Left) Father: Clayton Charles, Artist (Right) Grandfather: Clayton Charles, Surgeon

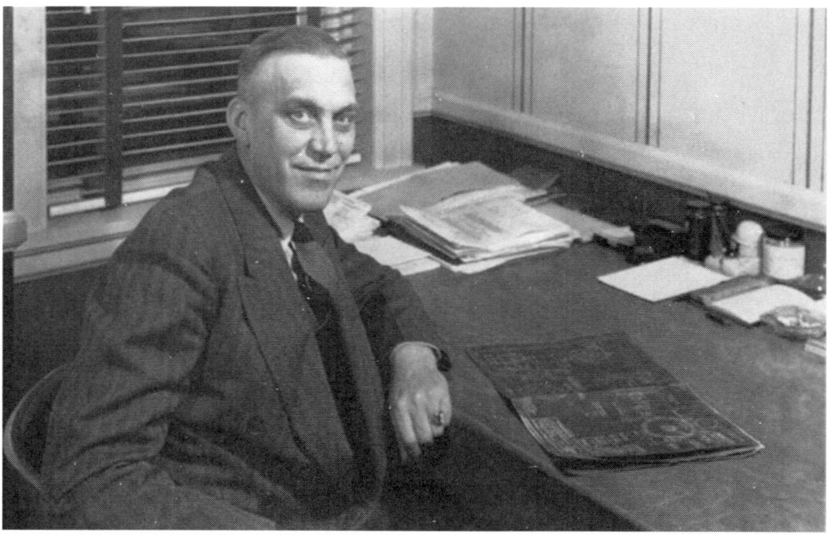

Maternal Grandfather: Harry Johnson, Mechanical Engineer

"I grew up in a house of ideas," Charles said. "We had people like poet Robert Frost over for dinner, and I can remember meeting Frank Lloyd Wright at his home in Madison, Wisconsin. I had dinner with Jacques Cousteau at my father's friend's home."

During the summer of 1969, Charles, athletic and fastidious to the point where specks of dirt on the floor were a distraction, was a medical student doing research. In Miami, he was working in the community where he had been raised and was energized by the fact that he had discovered his calling in eye surgery. Cataract operations somewhat bored him with simplicity, but the precision and intricacies of the human eye and its transformation of light to moving images was endlessly intriguing to him. He could not stop studying and performing practice surgeries on the eyes of lab animals as he contemplated better and more efficient methods for improving surgical techniques.

"I scrubbed in on a lot of different types of surgeries at the V.A. Hospital when I was a medical student," Charles said. "I saw surgeons draining abscesses, sectioning bowels, and it had no appeal to me. But the eye was something precise and beautiful. Anyone with an engineering mind or background would be drawn to what the eye does. I guess I really clicked with the ophthalmologists. I met all the super guys from Bascom Palmer in those years—Dave Sime, Danny Jones, Joel Glaser—and they let me assist on cataract surgery. They also gave me all their damaged instruments, and I fixed them. Sometimes I used the repaired instruments to do cataract surgery on dogs that were getting kidney transplants in the experimental surgery labs."

Two of the most important developments in the history of eye surgery were about to unfold at BPEI during Charles' years there. Ed Norton had convinced the Miami Kiwanis to create an eye bank for his physicians. The eye bank provided donated eyes for corneal transplants and ocular tissue for research, and Dr. Kasner, who had been teaching resident physicians how to perform cataract surgery, took full advantage of that resource.

Kasner, so thin and tall at six feet six inches that he always seemed to be leaning over to communicate, had installed air-conditioning in his home garage. He added a microscope, camera, lights, and dissection tables in order to study the anatomy of the front of the eye to improve outcomes for his cataract operations.

His surgeries, however, forced him to deal with the vitreous, because he was always entering the anterior (front) chamber of the eye. Unless the vitreous was removed, various side effects could result in visual loss when postoperative cataract complications occurred. Consequently, Kasner became the first American physician to intentionally and safely remove the vitreous. The idea was almost incomprehensible to previous generations of ophthalmologic surgeons, who believed that the eye was not likely to ever function properly without vitreous, though no science had proved that assertion.

"There were so many historically significant people and accomplishments at Bascom Palmer during those years, it is hard to measure the overall impact," said Kirk Packo, M.D., a Chicago retinal surgeon and historian of the evolution of the discipline. "This was the dawn of vitreous surgery, and there really is no way for us to know how many people see today because of developments at Bascom Palmer in the '60s and '70s. And Steve Charles was in the middle of all that."

Charles practically lived at BPEI and learned from residents like Sime and Jones, retinal fellows like Thomas Aaberg and Dennis Robertson, and faculty like Kasner as they performed ocular surgery. Kasner, in fact, often managed treatment of a major intraoperative complication that occurred after the removal of the eye's cloudy lens, which led to him taking a unique approach to treatment. Vitreous frequently migrated forward into the anterior chamber, causing detachment of the retina or creating cysts like macular edema (swelling) in the center of the retina, which resulted in the loss of central vision. A few different approaches had been attempted to keep vitreous out of the eye's front chamber with only limited positive results.

As early as 1961, Kasner had begun experimenting with removal of the vitreous from the eye using a new surgical technique he called "open sky." The procedure involved making a 300-degree incision in the cornea and then folding it open and back. (Picture an open toilet seat.) The doctor then reached into the exposed inner eye, engaged the vitreous with an absorbent cellulose sponge, carefully lifted a small portion, and used scissors to cut it loose from the remaining vitreous. The process was repeated until the remainder of the vitreous had fallen backward into the eye, behind the plane of the iris.

Kasner's goal was to prevent the vitreous from moving forward and contacting the cornea, which often caused swelling and vision loss, necessitating more surgery. The migration forward also had the potential to create traction on the retina in the back of the eye, which might pull it enough to cause a tear and detachment. Risks of open sky were not insignificant, and patients were rendered aphakic, a term that describes an eye that has undergone removal or loss of the natural lens. There was also the chance of hemorrhage and damage to the iris or cornea. Even the slightest excessive tug of the vitreous created traction and could pull the retina away from the wall of the eye, causing a retinal detachment that then would require surgery in an attempt to restore vision.

Kasner had become convinced, however, that vitreous could be safely removed from the eye, and he began to accumulate data to prove this. His initial open-sky operation involved an eight-year-old boy whose eye had been injured by a tent stake. The child's cornea had been cut, and material from the lens had broken loose and was retained in the vitreous space. On July 28, 1961, Kasner made a large incision to open the cornea, folded it back, and then used his sponge-and-scissors technique to remove the vitreous. Although the patient had been initially blinded by the accident, he retained a corrected vision of 20/50 decades after Kasner's repair surgery.

"Kasner had done something that we all thought was unheard of," said Robert Machemer decades later. "He had purposefully removed the vitreous from eyes. He said, 'I am not panicking anymore when the BPEI residents lose vitreous. I know you can remove it. Actually, you *have* to remove it. You will get better results.' And we were aghast. And we were more aghast when he, one day, reported about a patient where he had used what was called open-sky technique."

Kasner believed that removal of the vitreous was a solution to numerous pathological issues associated with the inner eye. In 1966 and '67, he operated on two patients who had developed opacity in the vitreous as a consequence of amyloidosis, which is a deposit of a pathologic protein. Kasner again did the corneal incision, lifted it back and folded it over, extracted the lens, and used cellulose sponges and scissors to lift and then cut the vitreous out of the eye, pulling the substance gingerly for each cut in order to avoid traction on the retina. The results were difficult to believe: One patient had been able to see only hand motions prior to the procedure and had 20/30 vision almost the next day. The other individual improved from 20/100 to 20/40. Just a few years earlier, both patients would have been told they had to live with the loss of visual acuity because medicine lacked effective treatment for their problems.

No one paid closer attention to Kasner's accomplishments than his BPEI colleague Robert Machemer. The German immigrant was determined to find a way to remove vitreous without the trauma of opening the front of the eye with a large incision. He had begun to contemplate taking a "pars plana" approach to entering the eye, creating an incision between the lens and retina, which enabled entry to the intraocular space without injuring the retina. Instead of lifting the cornea with a 300-degree wound, Machemer became confident vitreous might be cut and aspirated through the pars plana, if there were an appropriate instrument.

But none existed.

It seemed, in hindsight, almost providential that Jean-Marie Parel would meet Ed Norton at an international conference on Fluorescein Angiography in Albi, France, in 1969. The physicist had been dispatched by his university in Melbourne to a professional gathering about a technique for examining the circulation of the retina and the underlying choroid through the use of a fluorescent dye and a specialized angiography camera. When Parel met the kindly ophthalmologist from South Florida at the conference, he began a conversation that would lead him and his family to Miami.

Norton asked him what he had done in Australia, and the physicist presented the surgeon with a handwritten book of his drawings. The pages included sketches of what was to become known as the Vitreous Infusion Suction Cutter, or VISC. The early version derived from Parel's efforts to create micro-instruments for vascular operations; he had designed a vitreous band-cutter tip that had never been used in surgery. His next step was refining his drawings and offering a vision of the tool that would soon attract Machemer's interest.

"But it was really just a cutter," said Parel. "I didn't have any aspiration to get the vitreous out or any way to keep the pressure up in the eye. The idea we had in Australia was that you could go in and out. But after I met Robert Machemer, he made it clear we had to keep up the intraocular pressure because [otherwise] the eye would collapse, and we'd have a problem. We corresponded by mail, and I made the device and sent designs back to him for comments. Dr. Machemer liked the idea of keeping all the functions in one instrument to leave the other hand free."

Norton had urged Parel to turn his visit to the conference in France into an around-the-world trip with a stop in Miami to tour BPEI. Norton was interested in having his doctors, including the young engineer and medical student Steve Charles, get a look at some of Parel's designs. Always visionary, the Chief, as Norton was fondly called, wanted his staff thinking about microsurgical instruments. If wounds could be made smaller and less traumatic, surgical results could improve, and procedures were certain to become safer with purpose-built instrumentation that was reduced in size.

When Parel arrived in Miami, Machemer asked him what he was doing at BPEI, and when the German doctor saw the drawings of the vitreous tip cutter, he instantly focused on its potential to enter the eye without using open-sky incisions. Machemer and Parel went to lunch and made sketches on napkins. The Australian was later offered a job, and he returned home to prepare his student visa and rework his cutter-tool drawings.

Although Parel and Machemer exchanged designs and critiques by mail over the next months, the ambitious and taciturn Machemer was also impatient. He began work on a prototype VISC with researcher Helmet Buettner, M.D. The tool Machemer was using in the historical photograph of the egg was, in fact, that prototype—an airplane drill rotating in a stationary tube, a 30-cc plastic syringe with a small battery-driven motor. A second tube was soldered to the side to add suction, and when vitreous tissue was drawn into the hollow tube, the rotating drill cut it. Machemer used it successfully on a patient for an open-sky procedure and was encouraged by the results and the patient's cleared field of vision.

After Parel returned from Australia with the vitreous cutter he had built in his Melbourne lab, however, Machemer all but abandoned the invention he had developed with Buettner. He immediately recognized Parel as the engineering colleague he needed. Parel, though, had little time to assimilate to his new home. No sooner had he walked into BPEI with his wife and son in tow after the long trip from Australia then Machemer took them to a hotel a few blocks away, showed Mrs. Parel and the boy where to have lunch, and brought his new colleague back to the lab. There was no post-flight nap to combat jet lag, no civilized meal, no time to help his family settle in before getting down to work.

"Robert was the most impatient man on earth," Parel said. "You can imagine what it was like back in those days. I felt like it took about a week to get to Miami from Australia on an airplane, and then, a half-hour after the airplane lands, I was at Bascom Palmer. [Robert] said, 'I want to see the machine,' and we did in vitro testing right there that day. Two or three days later we did a rabbit, and a week later, we did a human being."

The historic surgery using the VISC was performed on April 20, 1970, at Jackson Memorial Hospital in Miami. The first human to experience a pars plana vitrectomy was a diabetic patient who had five years of visual opacity caused by hemorrhage inside the eye. According to Machemer, everyone had insisted nothing could be done to improve the man's vision. Before the operation, the patient saw only hand motions at a few feet. Machemer, however, used the VISC to enter the eye behind the lens without a large incision, cut and removed the bloody vitreous, and the man was almost immediately able to see with 20/40 vision.

"Such a result was totally unheard of before," Machemer said many years later during a forum. "This was like a bombshell at the time. But it was also in the air. I remember getting a letter from a soldier in Vietnam, who proposed a little propeller to liquefy vitreous to remove it. So ophthalmology, in a way, was ready to take on a problem that they still couldn't tackle. And I was lucky to be there at that time and to be stimulated by the faculty at Miami."

Parel immediately set to improving the VISC. He had already worked with Charles to manage the voltage and changes in the electrical power source to adapt them from Australian standards. He was also heeding Charles' advice that the instrument—especially the gauge, or width, of the inserted hollow needle that carried the cutting tool—should be smaller. Charles and others felt there needed to be a smaller incision on the eye's surface because a reduced wound size offers quicker recovery and less danger to the eye. Parel, Buettner, and Machemer were relying significantly on Charles, by now an intern, to provide them with mechanical guidance on various types of devices and instruments. Charles had been given office space on BPEI's fourth floor and had turned it into an engineering lab just a few doors down from Parel's office.

"For eight years of medical school, internship, and residency, I kept working on a variety of engineering projects," Charles said. "I significantly improved the electronics of the ERG [electroretinography] machine they had, built the first electro-oculography [EOG] machine—from dome to amplifiers to display screen—from scratch, improved the pupillography machine, and performed experimental retinal detachment surgery with Machemer. I don't think I could ever explain what an exciting time this was for all of us."

While Machemer was trying to improve the technique of pars plana vitrectomy, Parel and Buettner were making refinements in the mechanical efficiency and safety of the VISC.

Everyone at BPEI knew that a profound moment in ophthalmology had occurred when Robert Machemer completed the first successful PPV at Jackson Memorial Hospital in Miami. People with previously inoperable retinal conditions that caused blindness were now likely to be given positive results. The impact of the new surgical tool and techniques of pars plana vitrectomy remained incalculable.

THREE

Rotation Speed

Almost exactly 40 years after Machemer's advancement of retinal care, and still long before I met Steve Charles, I was in Austin, Texas, about to experience Machemer's innovative operation for myself. Dr. D's previous use of a laser in his office to repair my horseshoe-shaped retinal tear had failed. The tear broke loose in a few days, and vitreous began to move behind the retina, causing a detachment. Half of my field of vision in the right eye had already disappeared, as if a drape had been lowered across it.

I was as unaware as any other retinal patient of the work of Machemer, Parel, Charles, Buettner, Norton, and all the other researchers and physicians who had improved pars plana vitrectomy and given back eyesight to countless patients. I did, however, trust the science and technology of PPV surgery and the training, experience, and competency of my physician.

Dr. D always wore the same style of white coat that had been worn by the visionaries of his discipline, and he had been to the best schools, held professional board certifications, and had years of training and experience. He seemed serious and confident with a soft, reassuring voice, which, I suspect now, may have even lulled me into complacency.

My nature is to be skeptical, a characteristic acquired after decades as a journalist chasing politicians across the country and parsing their words for disingenuousness. I did not abandon my inquisitiveness or demand for information as I sat in Dr. D's exam chair, but I confess to believing in an American educational and training system that had delivered him to Austin, and he was dressed in that white coat, a symbol of a legacy of skill and competency.

But sometimes it was just a coat.

Dr. D reclined my exam chair and leaned over to peer into my dilated right eye. He used a head-worn indirect ophthalmoscope and handheld lens to examine the condition of my retina.

"We're going to need to go inside your eye to repair this," Dr. D said. "Your retina has detached."

"Going inside? I guess that means surgery?"

"Yes, you need a vitrectomy."

"Which is what, exactly?"

"We use tools to enter the eye and remove the vitreous and fluid behind the retina, and that allows the retina to return to the back wall of your eye," he said. "Then, we use laser inside the eye to ensure that it stays reattached, and we replace the vitreous with a solution or gas to create pressure to hold everything in place while it heals."

"That's a common procedure?"

"Yes, it's been successful for decades. I perform multiple vitrectomies every week."

"I assume the sooner the better?"

"Yes, we will schedule for surgery first thing tomorrow."

At the front desk, Dr. D told his assistant to schedule me for a pars plana vitrectomy, a phrase I was to hear many times. I had no idea what the procedure might involve and didn't bother to do my usual Internet search to learn. Every sentence from Dr. D made this sound routine. I was not overly concerned about any associated issues and certainly did not contemplate harm to my vision. I had been almost absurdly healthy for my 60 years, never missed work, and had been an endurance athlete as a competitive distance runner for more than half of my life. I assumed the operation would be successful, that I would heal fast, and my eyesight would quickly return to normal.

My detachment was classified as rhegmatogenous, a term that describes subretinal fluid moving into the space between the neurosensory retina and the underlying tissue, known as the retinal pigment epithelium (RPE). The RPE lines the scleral wall of the eye and is a cell layer just beyond the neurosensory retina. It is responsible for nourishing retinal visual cells and is attached to the underlying choroid—the location of blood veins—and the overlying visual cells of the retina. *Rhegma,* I discovered, was a Greek word that referred to a discontinuity or break, which is the most common type of retinal detachment. My surgery would involve a laser light inserted through a cannula, a hollow needle, punched through the pars plana at the front of the eye during the removal of the vitreous.

Using light with an instrument that functions in the interior of the eye by going through the scleral wall, rather than through the pupil, is a process called endo-photocoagulation. Steve Charles, who created the hybrid word, also developed the process as a young physician engineer in 1974.

Heat, cold, and light had been used historically, with various degrees of efficiency, to reattach the retina or to repair breaks. In the 1930s, a needle might be heated and poked through the eye at a location where the retina needed repairing. The heat caused tissue and blood proteins to coagulate at 65 °C. In the 1960s and after, a cold cryoprobe could also be used to achieve the same results: killing cells and causing a tiny spot of scar tissue called a chorioretinal adhesion that acted like a weld to hold the retina in position against the RPE lining the eye.

Prior to Charles' innovation, light was delivered for retinal repair by going through the pupil, a technique that had limited effectiveness for a number of reasons, including the constrained range of vision for doctors trying to see through the pupil, which, even after dilation, is still a narrow aperture. The biggest limitation was that light energy could not be applied to a *detached* retina; it had to be attached first.

Retinopexy, holding the retina in place to heal and prevent vision-threatening detachments, was increasingly achieved using light. However, the only tool for this procedure in the 1970s was a large and powerful light source known as the Zeiss photocoagulator. The light from the Zeiss box was created using xenon, a colorless, odorless, inert gas that delivers intensely bright and powerful illumination when properly activated.

An additional and early important purpose of the Zeiss photocoagulator was to stop the visual decay suffered by diabetic patients. The disease often causes the proliferative growth of small arterioles and capillaries along the retina. They tend to bleed as well as create scar tissue, which detaches the retina. Focused light from the Zeiss was used to cause the coagulation of retinal areas and abnormal blood vessels and stop the hemorrhages.

An outsize component of the Zeiss photocoagulator, almost like a proboscis, was used to send light through the pupil to the targeted spot, but it was relatively impractical because of the constant movement of the doctor's scope to adjust the visual field.

Charles disliked the Zeiss box for two reasons: He could not abide the requirement to first attach the retina, nor did he care for the tool's ergonomic and workspace limitations.

"I just thought, after using this big box so many times, that I needed to send the light into the eye using a fiber bundle," he said. "This wasn't really a eureka kind of thing. It just struck me as logical. I had a problem and thought up a way to solve it. But I also knew as you took the light into these narrow fiber bundles, the heat would be concentrated. I needed a way to manage the heat."

A high temperature would make the device dangerous to both the operator and the patient and jeopardize the reliability of Charles' idea. To lower the heat, he attached a series of metal fins at the junction of the Zeiss to the fiber bundle and then used a vacuum to draw air across the fins and dissipate the heat. The resulting tiny fiber bundle was inserted into a blunt metal needle that could be pushed through the scleral wall at the pars plana. That put light-induced heat precisely where it was intended, while the physician controlled the tool's movements. The efficiency and overall effectiveness of light repair for retinal holes, breaks, tears, and diabetic retinopathy was now greatly improved.

Endo-photocoagulation was Charles' first significant engineering idea, and it began his long career of transforming the new medical subspecialty known as vitreoretinal surgery. Although Charles' advancement of eye treatment using fiber optics was reported in peer-reviewed medical literature, two other physicians claimed to have invented it several years later.

Charles was to discover claims like those are not unusual. Because he was more inclined to treat patients, innovate, and teach instead of write scientific papers for universities, he had to contend with the problem of others trying to put their name on his accomplishments.

Throughout the course of his long career of surgery and invention, the doctor has mostly refrained from expending energy on writing for professional publications and waiting months for peer reviews. He likes to solve problems, not write about them in the quotable peer-reviewed literature, which can lead to others claiming similar achievements. Inevitably, controversies arose related to credit for inventing and improving techniques, an occurrence that has been intertwined with the evolution of medicine. Ideas that might be considered obvious often occur to more than one person when treatment reaches a certain point of scientific sophistication. Without diligent documentation and peer review, pretenders can claim to have reached a milestone first.

Even with publication in professional journals, though, conflicts can arise over the origination of an invention, as others at BPEI found. David Kasner, for instance, is remembered as the surgeon who developed open-sky approaches to the vitreous in the eye, which he detailed in his 1968 paper. Seventeen years earlier, however, Dr. Tsugio Dodo, a Japanese physician, had already performed the operation in precisely the same manner at a Hiroshima hospital.

Dodo's work was published in a Japanese journal and included pictures that reflected the same technique explained in Kasner's paper. Medical history appears to have given Kasner full credit for the process, though, in part because he relentlessly spread his idea. Meanwhile, Western physicians knew little or nothing of Dodo's successes in Japan. Dr. Kasner probably had no idea about the work of Dr. Tsugio Dodo, reported in the Japanese language on the other side of the world, long before the Internet might have spread unique thinking or left ideas and intellectual property largely unprotected.

Observing the trauma and dangers associated with cutting the front of the eye in open-sky operations intensified Robert Machemer's interest in a closed vitrectomy procedure. But he, too, had been preceded by another Japanese surgeon. Machemer, who was almost certainly oblivious to the innovation he was to duplicate and refine, was more than a decade behind physician and inventor Dr. Chouzapurou Haruta in Osaka. The Japanese doctor performed the first documented closed vitrectomy—though technically it was not a vitrectomy since he did not remove the vitreous—in 1959, and his work was widely published in Japanese journals.

Machemer's celebrated operation in Miami did not occur until 1970.

Haruta relied on cryotherapy: Using a cryoprobe on the outside of the eye, he essentially created scar tissue by freezing the retina at precise locations to keep it reattached. Scar tissue created by freezing externally is similar to the coagulation that occurs when using laser internally. Haruta was able to treat problems with the vitreous using the cryoprobe without entering the eye through the surgically opened cornea or puncturing the adjacent pars plana.

Almost a half century after Machemer performed what is considered the first pars plana vitrectomy, his legacy has become even cloudier. Anton Banko, a mechanical engineer in New York City, was laboring in relative obscurity at a dental device company, developing the fluidics in ultrasonic technology for cleaning teeth, when an ophthalmologist approached him about a concept for removing cataracts. During a dental appointment, Dr. Charles Kelman was struck by the thought that high-speed vibrations might be employed in a handheld tool to emulsify cataract-clouded lenses without surgical excision. Kelman and Banko collaborated on a mechanical means of removing the lens, which led, eventually, to the modern procedure known as phacoemulsification, used in removing cataracts and, ultimately, the insertion of clear, artificial lenses. Banko developed the fluidics for the initial phacoemulsification machine, a procedure that is appropriately credited to Kelman. The high-speed vibrations that Kelman had experienced getting his teeth cleaned had been used to emulsify clouded lenses, which made their removal considerably safer through a small incision.

Banko also began a professional association with Dr. Charles Schepens of Harvard Medical School. Schepens, a Belgian immigrant to the United States after World War II, is recognized as the creator of the retinal subspecialty of ophthalmology. As founder of the world's first treatment center for the retina in 1949, Schepens was a pioneer who was equally well known for importing the binocular indirect ophthalmoscope to the U.S., where it is used routinely, as it is in the rest of the world, to examine the retina.

There is no way to identify the source of another of Banko's ideas, but it seems likely his association with Kelman and Schepens prompted him to contemplate a solution to a difficult problem regarding eye surgery. At some point before 1968, Anton Banko began work on an electrical device to cut and aspirate vitreous from the human eye. His company, Surgical Design, filed a patent for a tool that performed the same tasks as the Vitreous Infusion Suction Cutter (VISC) developed by Machemer and Jean-Marie Parel. In the language of the patent office, it was: "Apparatus for Performing Surgical Procedures on the Eye. U.S. Patent No. 3,528,425; filed on September 16, 1968 and patented September 15, 1970."

Machemer never sought a patent for the VISC, and he did not perform his first vitrectomy with the tool until April 20, 1970, about 19 months after Banko had filed his paperwork with the federal government. Neither a doctor nor an educator, Banko was an engineer who "made things;" he was not ideally suited to spreading the news of his work or to promote his ideas. However, Schepens described Banko's work in great detail and insisted the instrument to perform vitreoretinal closed surgeries existed well before Machemer's initial use of the VISC. Schepens and Banko reportedly conducted numerous operations with his device at the Retina Foundation of Boston under the auspices of Harvard University.

In fact, there's a possibility that Machemer's idea may have been subtly expropriated from Banko, though most medical historians insist that Parel and Machemer conceived and created the VISC with only their inspiration and education. Banko's son, though, had called and written a letter to Ed Norton, inquiring if the facility could make use of his father's invention, which was described as a "vitrectomy cutter with aspiration and coaxial fusion." The logical conclusion is that if such a letter were indeed delivered, Norton would have shared the information with Machemer, a man he knew to be obsessed with finding a way to remove vitreous without large corneal incisions.

"It's pretty much inescapable that the Banko drawings in his patent application look really similar to the VISC," said medical historian Kirk Packo. "And his abstract described it as a tool for removing foreign objects from the eye as well as blood clots and lens material. But I'm fairly certain this went through a U.S. patent court, and Machemer was cleared of any suspicions around theft of ideas. They concluded both tools were developed in parallel, and Machemer didn't have knowledge of Banko's machine."

Steve Charles was a medical student at the University of Miami and researcher at Bascom Palmer Eye Institute when Machemer arrived from Germany. Charles had assisted on enough cataract surgeries to know that he found them relatively boring and decidedly routine, even though the procedure was evolving with intraocular plastic lenses to return sight to previously unattained levels of acuity. When Jean-Marie Parel brought his prototype VISC to BPEI,

Charles was intrigued by both the mechanical and surgical possibilities for repairing retinas with an entirely new procedure. Machemer taught Charles how to perform a vitrectomy with the VISC and then allowed him to assist on surgeries while also encouraging him to refine his skills and teach.

"I know that people talk about this question of where the idea for the VISC originated," Charles said, "but I think that's almost irrelevant now. What we do know of Machemer is that he was a great surgeon, he was passionate, and he wrote widely and taught me—and any number of other young surgeons—how to do vitrectomies and do them successfully. He promoted the VISC and vitrectomy, and there is no question he's the reason it became an important ophthalmic subspecialty."

Nonetheless, as the VISC began to be widely used, a certain amount of antipathy developed between Machemer and Schepens. The Harvard ophthalmologist's stature as founder of the Retina Foundation in Boston meant he understood the importance and potential value of Banko's invention. According to Packo, Machemer threatened Schepens with a lawsuit when he was presented with Banko's vitreous cutter.

"Machemer was at Duke for a presentation," Packo explained. "And Schepens came out with this thing that Banko had made, and it looked identical to the VISC. Machemer said he'd sue him if [Schepens] tried to commercialize this. It was really clear that Schepens and Machemer didn't get along."

For his part, Parel considered any close association between Schepens and Banko improbable, because Schepens resisted using the pars plana for vitrectomies. Parel noted that during a presentation to a thousand ophthalmologists at the American Academy of Ophthalmology and Otolaryngology, Machemer had offered data on the success rates of vitrectomies using his new technique, which was praised by the physicians there. Less than an hour later, Schepens took to the podium to say that pars plana would harm the eyes and that open sky was the best way to do a vitrectomy.

"So I can't imagine Banko working with Schepens on a VISC," Parel said. "It doesn't make any sense. But Banko, one day, decided to accuse the University of Miami of stealing his ideas and violating his patents. It was misguided. The lawyers saw that we had the documents to show that we had done it before he did. We won that war."

No evidence, in fact, ever surfaced to show any linkage between Banko's drawings and Machemer's and Parel's work on the VISC.

With the passage of time, what really happened is probably unknowable. We are left with the importance of what *definitely did* transpire: Machemer and BPEI actively promoted and taught vitreoretinal surgery with the VISC. Machemer had at his disposal BPEI's expanding reputation and resources. He was a gifted and ambitious surgeon determined to share with his profession the excitement of a new tool and technique for saving damaged retinas and eyesight, and that's what he did with great enthusiasm. Eventually, after a 12-year tenure at BPEI, he became the chairman of Duke University's Department of Ophthalmology, where he was described by colleagues as "an excellent clinician, a tremendous educator, and a wonderful researcher."

"With the development of mechanized vitreous aspiration and cutting, which Dr. Machemer introduced, we were exposed to an entirely new field within our discipline," said Priscilla E. Perry, M.D., associate clinical professor at Louisiana State University School of Medicine, Shreveport. "Prior to this time, there was no controlled way to handle vitreous disease and the associated retinal pathology."

These foundational changes in eye surgery were occurring while

Steve Charles was studying at BPEI. The Chief had taken Charles under his wing, given him his first indirect ophthalmoscope at the beginning of his second year in medical school, and even sought his insights on research. Norton's children suffered from retinitis pigmentosa, a progressive deterioration of vision caused by the death of the retina's rods and cones, the photoreceptor cells that gather light to deliver moving images to the brain; Charles was working on the causes of the death of rods and cones in the human eye and the resulting diminishment of vision. Norton often scheduled after-hours meetings with Charles to discuss their findings in electroretinography (ERG), an electrical test to measure retinal function.

Charles' intense determination as a medical student was obvious and made an impression on those around him. When Norton offered Charles a residency at BPEI, Victor Curtin, the institute's first faculty member—who would serve 57 years—offered Charles money for his schoolbooks. Charles was unafraid of any kind of work that helped cover his expenses. The week before he began medical school, he was making extra money using a power saw to cut away fallen trees after hurricanes. He spent his first year of medical school living at the V.A. Hospital in Coral Gables, beginning his workdays with blood draws at five a.m. He scrubbed in with any doctor willing to let him into an operating room.

"When I couldn't get into the operating room, I would perform experimental surgery in the lab. I watched the ophthalmology residents, as well as ear, nose, and throat and the neurosurgeons every chance I had. As a senior medical student, I went to the lab at night and stuck electrodes in cats' brains. Then, later at night, I went over to the undergraduate campus and studied engineering."

Charles also watched with great interest the evolution of vitrectomy surgery at BPEI and the improvements to the VISC. The final version of that tool had included a coaxial line to infuse saline to maintain eye pressure as the vitreous was cut and sucked outward through a separate, parallel small tube. Without pressure, the eye would collapse, and Machemer had previously managed this by using a needle to inject air or fluid. Parel later added a fiber optic endo-illuminator to the tip of the cutter, which enabled surgeons to see in the intraocular space without having to shine a light through the pupil.

Parel and Dr. Helmet Buettner were also consistently present when Robert Machemer was performing vitrectomies, and they concentrated on improving technical aspects while keeping the VISC functional with any needed repairs. Charles had always thought the VISC—especially the gauge of the needle tube inserted into the eye—was too large. And he did not like the fact that the vacuum to remove fluid from the eye was controlled by an assistant using a hand syringe. He thought that should be done by the surgeon.

Charles had been doing experimental retinal detachment surgery with Machemer, and he increased his training in vitrectomy using the VISC. He also had the opportunity to do about 90 scleral buckle operations, a technique that involved sewing a type of rubber band around the eye to change the interior pressure and hold a detached retina against the sclera so it could heal. Charles' time in the operating room also increased when Norton and Dr. Donald Gass of the BPEI faculty had too many commitments to perform their normal quotient of surgeries. The young man used circumstances like that to his advantage.

After Charles' years of medical school, internship, and residency at BPEI, fellow trainees and the faculty recognized his diligence and skill. The Chief, in fact, had begun conversations with Carl Kupfer, director of the National Eye Institute (NEI) near Washington, D.C., about Charles' idea of using vitrectomy to search for angiogenic factors, which are molecules that exert a fundamental role in the formation of blood vessels. Charles was a natural choice for the program because of the time he'd spent in surgeries with Machemer and his knowledge of the VISC. He was also interested in trying to prove the existence of something called the Vascular Proliferative Factor (VPF), the angiogenic material that researchers theorized prompted the body to grow abnormal blood vessels.

There were two positions in the NEI program, and hundreds of young ophthalmologists applied. Charles was rewarded with one of the spots.

On his last day at BPEI, Charles walked through the front lobby to the main door. He had to pass a huge mosaic along the wall. "The Woman at the Window" had been chosen for the display by the young physician's father when art was commissioned for the building. The Chief was out of the building when Charles was making his rounds to say good-bye. But, at the last minute, the two men crossed paths. At that moment, the young surgeon found himself standing between the artwork admired by his father, chairman of the University of Miami's Department of Art, and in front of his mentor. Both men had given him the guidance and wisdom needed to achieve excellence in medicine.

"Dr. Norton," Steve Charles said, "what can I ever do to repay you for all you've done for me?"

Norton's Irish smile snapped into a gentle recognition, and he placed a hand on his student's shoulder.

"Teach," Norton said.

"I will, sir," Charles said. "I will."

Charles shook Norton's hand and then walked out into the South Florida sun, bound for Bethesda, Maryland. What lay before Steve Charles was far greater than even his eager mind might have imagined.

FOUR

A Portrait of the Doctor as a Young Man

He remembers the eyes.

A man who has operated on tens of thousands of people can hardly be expected to recall most of his patients and their names, but the eyes remain blazed in his memory. He sees the macular holes, the giant retinal breaks hanging like blown canvas, horseshoe tears, diabetic bleeding, epimacular membranes that need peeling from the retina's surface. He remembers how he arrived at decisions for treatment. Each eye taught him something, helped him become a better surgeon or a more innovative engineer, and, consequently, made it more likely that someone with a similar problem might not lose vision.

Around 1973, Steve Charles was operating at the National Eye Institute (NEI), under the purview of the National Institutes of Health (NIH) in Bethesda, Maryland, and was preparing a corneal transplant for a patient. The doctor had married and the first two of his three daughters had been born when he moved his young family to the Washington, D.C. area. He had been selected to begin the search for the Vascular Proliferative Factor (VPF), later called Vascular Endothelial Growth Factor (VEGF). Researchers increasingly believed a chemical response in the human body prompted the growth of tiny arteries and capillaries. If identified, it might be controlled, improving the odds of saving vision or even slowing cancer development.

On this morning, early in his NEI tenure, Charles was treating a patient with a cloudy cornea and cataract. He had already removed the corneal button with a trephine, a circular knife. A transplant cornea was at hand, but because the interior of the eye had been exposed, Charles looked inside to make certain there were no other complications. After removing the cataract, the doctor saw a vitreous hemorrhage that needed to be removed. The bleeding into the vitreous was certain to impair the patient's future vision. Using a new vitreous cutter known as a Roto-Extractor, Charles excised the vitreous and then discovered a large detachment with a hole in the retina.

After only six months, the NEI had switched from Machemer and Parel's VISC to the Roto-Extractor, which had been designed and built by Nicholas Douvas, a cataract surgeon in Port Huron, Michigan. Douvas had developed his cutter soon after Machemer in 1968 but for a different purpose: Douvas needed a way to remove hardened, or fibrotic, cataracts to prevent them from causing damage at the front of the eye or moving into the vitreous to create complications that might lead to a retinal detachment. The Roto-Extractor also used a multi-turn oscillatory cutting mode that somewhat reduced the problem of vitreous winding with the VISC. Vitreous collagen fibers often wrapped around the rotating cutter and could pull on the retina and cause detachments. Douvas' device reduced that probability.

That morning, at NEI, Charles noticed that fluid had migrated through the patient's retinal hole and was accumulating under the retina. The fluid had to be removed to enable reattachment of the retina to the retinal pigment epithelium (RPE), the cellular layer that provides nourishment to the light-sensitive retinal tissue. Standard practice since the inception of retinal detachment surgery was to externally cut through the scleral wall of the eye and drain the subretinal fluid from the outside, a procedure known as a drainage or cut down sclerotomy. This allowed the retina to move back into position after the fluid had been drained through the incision. Unfortunately, sclerotomy was not a perfect procedure, because all the fluid behind the retina could not always be drained. Retinal entrapment often occurred in the sclerotomy, along with, on occasion, hemorrhage from the layer of blood vessels called the choroid.

In this case, Charles thought that he ought to try placing the tip of the Roto-Extractor through the hole and use it to remove the subretinal fluid. As he withdrew the fluid through the extractor, the retina began to move back into place in the patient's eye. Charles pulled on the syringe portion of the extractor after he had turned off the cutting function, and the subretinal fluid was slowly sucked out. The retina returned to its proper position against the RPE. Charles had just invented a process known as internal drainage of subretinal fluid, and it remains the standard of care after more than 40 years. No one had previously considered draining fluid through an extant hole in a detached retina, undoubtedly because they were fearful of complications.

"What's the meaning of this?" Charles asked from a vantage point that was years removed from that morning in the NEI operating room. "I always want to know how developments fit into the process of innovation. This occurred to me on the spot in the OR. I said, 'Wait a minute. This isn't about publishing a paper.' I just asked why are they making a hole in the sclera and draining from the outside. There is always a risk of bleeding if you cut through the eye wall. This way, we avoid choroidal hemorrhage, and we drain all the fluid without catching retina in the incision. Risk is reduced."

Invention is often the product of an idea cascade. Creation of one tool or methodology can open new thinking regarding other barriers blocking optimal functionality. Because he was bright, insightful, and driven, Charles understood almost instinctively that his learning about the new surgical technique was far from concluded, which is what led to a series of new retinal concepts during his tenure working for the federal government. And although he realized he was improving the vitrectomy process, Charles could not know the far-reaching consequences of what he viewed as nothing more than his basic problem-solving skills.

Charles did not constrain himself and his interests at NEI any more than he had at BPEI. Instead of grabbing a few extra hours of sleep in the morning, Steve got up at 5:00 a.m. and headed for the Biomedical Engineering and Instrumentation Branch (BEIB) of NIH to design and build instruments he hoped would improve retinal surgery. He had no mandate from his supervisors, and the government would own whatever he invented, but every time the young surgeon confronted a problem, his mind raced to an engineering or methodological solution. He was not about to ignore advancements he could make to ophthalmology, especially to vitrectomy.

The actual purpose of Charles' engagement at NEI, however, was to look for VPF, the unidentified protein or molecule that prompted the body to grow new blood vessels on the retinal surface, iris, and the trabecular meshwork (the tissue around the base of the cornea responsible for draining the aqueous humor from the eye through the anterior chamber). It was thought that VPF caused leaking of serum from preexisting blood vessels in the eye, which resulted in a condition called diabetic macular edema or nonproliferative diabetic retinopathy. The growth of new blood vessels caused by the then-unidentified VPF/VEGF also led to bleeding and traction retinal detachment, referred to as proliferative diabetic retinopathy, which often necessitated vitrectomy.

Scientists understood that the lack of a sufficient oxygen supply to the retina in diabetics caused the capillaries to leak, but they had no idea what signaled the body to begin neovascularization in its attempt to save the retina. (The process of growing new blood vessels anywhere in the body is called angiogenesis, or neovascularization.) Diabetics can also lose vision because of nonproliferative retinopathy, but it is the almost uncontrolled intrusion of new blood vessels that tends to cause hemorrhage and scarring, which is related to traction retinal detachment and blindness.

In certain cases of vitrectomy on diabetic patients, Charles collected aspirates from the vitreous of patients with diabetic retinopathy. As experimental controls, he used aspirates from others with proliferative vitreoretinopathy (PVR), which is the movement and proliferation of the retinal pigment epithelium, or RPE cells, and glial cells, the providers of oxygen and nutrients to the retina. They create a fibrotic membrane during migration onto the surface of the vitreous cavity and the retina. This occurs after a previous retinal detachment surgery and has the same biological characteristics as excessive wound healing, but it causes these membranes to contract and pull on the retina, which leads to a secondary detachment.

The aspirates Charles used in his experiment were vitreous tissue that he had removed via the Roto-Extractor from within the intraocular chamber. Researchers thought there might be biological information in the aspirates that could be identified and then somehow stopped from signaling the body to grow abnormal blood vessels in the eye. They might, eventually, be used to create a drug or antibody to prevent diabetic blindness.

Charles came very close to another historic retinal breakthrough.

"We injected processed vitreous from the vitreous of a diabetic patient into a rhesus monkey eye," he said. "The iris actually did develop neovascularization, but because there was no ectropion uvea, the NEI pathologist was skeptical, and the study never got published. Nevertheless, I basically satisfied the postulate for VEGF without the ability to sequence it, which was pretty cool in hindsight."

Ectropion uvea was considered an important indicator of iris neovascularization, although it was actually a late complication. Researchers thought that there would be eversion, a turning outward of the pigmented posterior epithelium cells near the margin of the pupil, if a molecule were prompting neovascularization. The fact that did not happen in Charles' VEGF experiments with monkeys kept him from receiving credit for identifying what was later determined by others to be VEGF. But the vitreous aspirates had caused blood-vessel growth in the eyes of the rhesus; consequently, there was no denying that a substance within the vitreous was causing neovascularization.

Science can often move as slowly as the worst bureaucracies. And it was a bureaucratic failure that may have delayed the ultimate identification of VEGF. Charles, though, was busy with multiple other projects related to vitreoretinal surgery. In retrospect, a few of his ideas are so logical as to appear either brilliant or mundane. Charles was using the Roto-Extractor to perform his first internal drainage of subretinal fluid, when he thought that a hollow needle might be the simplest and best tool to accomplish fluid removal.

He designed a straight, hollow needle without a point, called a cannula, tapered at the end, to reach through the retinal hole or the tear with a syringe to withdraw the fluid that was causing the detachment. Eventually, Charles conceived the idea of a flute cannula, a 20-gauge pipe with a tapered tip that made insertion through a retinal break to drain subretinal fluid easier, using a finger-controlled port to control the removal of fluid.

By sharing his approach with other surgeons, Charles changed the technique for draining fluid, a process that used to require an incision in the sclera and choroid behind the detachment, where the fluid was accumulating. Although he had nothing to do with naming it, the flute cannula is still known as the "Charles Needle." Charles no longer uses his invention because a technique called extrusion—developed by California eye surgeon Conor O'Malley—eventually offered foot-pedal control.

Another widely recognized use of a cannula was to insert small, precise instruments into the eye to perform operations through the hollow tube. That was the product of the inventive mind of Dyson Hickingbotham, an engineer who worked at Duke University and later at top ocular instrument companies.

Charles, meanwhile, was doing what he was commissioned to do when he was accepted to the NEI program. Actually, he was accomplishing considerably more than had been expected. In addition to training doctors on vitrectomy, he was designing instruments, conducting research to identify VEGF, and speaking to physicians' groups. In fact, a Georgetown University retinal surgeon, who often came to NEI to watch Charles work, asked the young doctor to speak on diabetic traction retinal detachment. The seemingly harmless invitation ended with the doctor being banned from the operating room at NEI for many agonizing months.

"I got summoned to the director's office," Charles explained. "He viewed it almost as the Oval Office. He was a big Nixon guy and made me sit at the end of a 15-foot table. He was angry with me for accepting a speaking invitation without his approval of my presentation. I was no longer allowed in the OR or the animal labs for months and months. It was ridiculous."

Charles found a way to subtly get revenge. As he walked to work, he made a point of cutting through the animal shelter where the NEI director, Carl Kupfer, housed monkeys he had brought from Seattle for glaucoma research. Charles secretly taught the monkeys to make an ugly gesture, undoubtedly to deliver a message to his boss the next time Kupfer came to the lab to conduct his experiments.

Charles rarely spent his hours frivolously, however. He had begun thinking about acquiring real-time images with ultrasound. Generally, a doctor used an ultrasonic scanning probe against the eyelid to take snapshots, which were examined to understand the pathology of a patient's case. B-scan ultrasound-imaging systems would send an ultrasonic beam along a plane or slice to capture a reflective image. The returned sound waves were turned into an image that was neither gray scale nor in real time. Both gray-scale and live images, however, gave a surgeon a better idea of each patient's situation. A gray scale meant that tissue densities were displayed as more or less white on a black screen and had the potential to show subtleties in the retina and vitreous that would be missed by a white or black non-gray-scale image.

"So, what was the notion behind this?" Charles asked. "By making it real time and gray scale, instead of black and white, you've created an alternative ophthalmoscope. Ultrasound scanning in real time allows me to look at a screen and get an idea of acoustic density as well as mobility and stiffness of tissue to distinguish a detached retina from vitreous hemorrhage, for example."

When Charles suggested to ultrasound companies the value of

a live, gray-scale, moving image of the intraocular space, he was informed such a thing was impossible. Jim Griffith, a brilliant engineer at the NIH instrumentation branch, however, eventually agreed to build the real-time imaging machine on Charles' specifications. The first time Charles put it against an eye, it worked beautifully and provided great live imagery. The real-time, gray-scale B-scan has changed little since the original was engineered in the early 1970s, and it remains a critical asset in the assessment of patients before vitreoretinal surgery. The motion on the screen helps doctors avoid reaching wrong conclusions before operating. In addition, sampling error is reduced, and tissue thickness and movement can be assessed with accuracy.

The technology was acquired by Xenotec and proved a valuable product for that company, but Charles made no money from it because he had developed it while working for the government. The instrumentation is used daily around the world without Charles' name attached, and few know who created such significant technology.

Charles' motivation was never profit or invention for its own sake. He has always been drawn to complex challenges to see if he can design a solution. Because the VISC and vitrectomy had created an entire surgical subspecialty, Charles discovered an opportunity to refine the new surgery with various inventions and techniques.

When he arrived at NEI in the middle of summer in 1973, he began a cycle of innovation that was to dramatically improve vitrectomy and its outcomes. During his two years in Washington, Charles devised 11 new technologies and techniques for improving retinal care during vitrectomy. These results may have been the consequence of his supervisor's banning him from the operating room and animal labs for months, which forced the surgeon to hang out at the engineering labs at NIH.

Once back in the operating room, however, Charles began to apply his insights and logic to the challenges presented by retinal damage, particularly detachment, often by trying out new tools he had just devised. The cannula that he had used to put through retinal holes and draw out fluid gave him another idea to improve the efficacy of this process. A coaxial cannula—two tubes placed one inside the other, with one opening slightly higher—allowed retinal fluid to be drained through one tube as air was infused into the eye through the other. The air supply was needed to restore surface tension and return the retina to its proper location. This helped keep up intraocular pressure so the eye would not collapse. This procedure, dubbed "fluid-air exchange," was quickly adopted throughout the vitreoretinal surgical community and has been a staple procedure throughout the modern era.

The other protocol, depending on the pathology of the patient's eye at the time of surgery, is the air-gas exchange. It, too, was also pioneered by Charles during his NEI service. Gas, usually perfluoropropane or sulfur hexafluoride, is mixed with air to eliminate expansive properties and is injected into the former vitreous cavity after the vitreous is removed. The air-gas mixture lasts longer than air alone and prevents fluid from flowing through retinal breaks. The air-gas mixture, which often requires a patient to lie facedown, floats against the retina in the posterior segment of the eye and provides surface tension to seal tears until the treated retinal breaks become bonded to the RPE. Charles' protocol followed work by Ed Norton and New York ophthalmologist Dr. Harvey Lincoff, who brought gas to the retinal community, and Dr. Gary Abrams of Detroit, who came up with the key concept of iso-expansive mixtures of air and gas.

In retrospect, these developments seem logical to practicing vitreoretinal surgeons, but at the time of conception, they were probably considered as risky as the first vitrectomy, especially since they came from the mind of a doctor who was barely 30. At 75, Steve Charles still inspires awe and a kind of stunned disbelief as you listen to his critical insights or watch him move through a room full of people. Charles pilots a high-performance business jet aircraft, exercises almost tirelessly, writes clearly about complex surgical concepts, and does all this with a level of energy that appears to exceed that of colleagues half his age. His schedule is rigorous and almost brutal by design: early morning exercise, surgeries, dozens of patients, travel to lectures or surgical demonstrations, engineering consulting with Alcon Laboratories. People who know the doctor well are often compelled to turn to religion to explain the arc of Steve Charles' life and his unrelenting push to heal, learn, and teach.

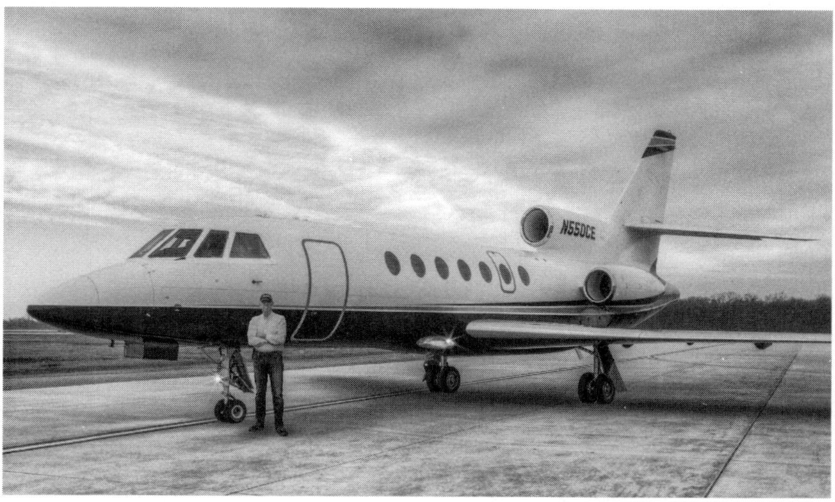

Charles and his Falcon 50 jet

There is more than a touch of irony in the fact that Charles, who lives a secular life and makes no private or public embrace of religion, tends to inspire spiritual explanations of his capabilities. John

Kevin Holbrook, a district judge in Kentucky, was sent to Charles' Retina Institute because his hometown surgeon was unable to repair a recurring detachment. Holbrook, who had already surrendered to the notion that his eye had been rendered permanently blind, left Memphis and headed home with nearly perfect vision, a new mentor, and a mystery.

"In the greater scheme of things," said Holbrook, who grew up in evangelical country, "I believe everything happens for a reason. And I had to come to know Dr. Charles for me to become the person God intended me to become. Now, I can't imagine my life without having this outstanding person in it. To have him know me personally, give me advice, and support me is one of the greatest honors I could be given. I can only hope I've given something to him in return. I've tried to explain to others what a truly remarkable person he is, but unless you've interacted with him personally, I suppose it's difficult to appreciate. I think God put him on this earth for reasons none of us can fully understand."

These are the types of sentiments Steve Charles has rarely taken the time to contemplate. Nor does he have any inclination for distracting introspection. If pressed for a belief system, the doctor invariably answers that he believes in "hard work, science, and love." There is always work to be done, something he has not thought about, an improvement for a process, or a new procedure or instrument. But Charles has no tendency to waste time looking for acclaim or plaudits. If he had been less inclined toward practical problem solving and more interested in writing academic papers, he might have had the medical profession and researchers singing his name to historians. Charles remains more pragmatic, however, and has chosen to spend his time understanding, fixing, and teaching.

"He could not bear the wasted time of superfluous publication," said Robert Laborde, M.D., a vitreoretinal surgeon and former fellow at the Charles Retina Institute. "So many academics employ Ph.D. candidates and fellows to churn out drivel that just doesn't advance the field of retina care. Steve would much rather design something, test it, advance it, and help patients with it, than sludge through the traditional channels of academia. The guy has vision and energy and technical skills, and at the same time he manages a super busy clinical load. There is just no time for the BS that academia demands."

Charles filled his rare spare moments in Washington by designing machines. Looking through the microscope into the eye during surgeries at NEI, he found it distracting to have to use a foot pedal to adjust the position of the microscope or the focus. The XY motor-drive box, which had been invented by Robert Machemer and Jean-Marie Parel, moved the microscope backward and forward and left and right, but Charles wanted to use the foot controls of the microscope to not only focus but also manage surgical functions like vacuum control. He resolved the issue by designing a chin switch that was attached to the microscope and provided excellent control without a foot pedal. Word got around in the retinal community, and Morgan Instruments built and sold 300 of his chin switches in a short period of time.

One of the other issues during those early days of vitrectomy surgery was the flow of fluid into and out of the eye. Machemer had managed this process by having an assistant operate a syringe. But a surgeon would be better able to assess the speed and amount of fluid needed to fill the inner eye. Charles designed a syringe drive—a hand wheel driving a rack and pinion to move the syringe plunger—that allowed a surgeon to smoothly control fluid aspiration.

With invention, innovation, and learning, Steve Charles' two years at NEI passed quickly. He had little time to contemplate the next step in his career or his future beyond that. Charles had met a few other retinal specialists through NEI, and he understood he had opportunities to join a large practice or open his own office. There was also the possibility of a university appointment and a life of research. The decision was hardly simple. It would certainly determine the course of the young doctor's life and that of his family.

Oddly, his early choice of business partner turned out to be a mistake, a rare and troubling experience for a young doctor unaccustomed to failure. But that choice pointed him to a city that would become his home.

FIVE

Patient One

We had no money, and I was embarrassed. A company I had been consulting for had previously placed me on their payroll, which made me eligible for their health-care plan, but after a relationship of several years, they had decided my services were no longer relevant to their business. My wife, Mary Lou, and I began to make payments to COBRA for continuation of benefits. The monthly total was around $2,000 and required a $5,000 deductible to get that "reduced" rate.

While I was being processed for retina surgery, the accounting clerk asked for my health-care card, punched numbers into her computer, and then looked up at me curiously.

"How would you like to take care of your portion of the surgical bill today?" she asked brightly, as if she were giving us a great opportunity.

"I guess I will decide that when I know how much it is."

"You'll need to cover your deductible, sir, which I see is $5,000. Your insurance will pick up the rest of the hospital's costs today."

"It's more than that?"

"Yes, the total bill is around $8,000 for use of the facilities. That doesn't cover your doctors, however."

"But I'm an outpatient. I'm going home."

"I understand."

"We have half of that in our checking account, I think," said Mary Lou, who had accompanied me. "I assume we can do the other half on a credit card?"

"Yes, ma'am, that will be fine."

As my bride of 35 years took care of the billing, my mind suddenly wandered to sunny Arizona and autumn baseball. My teammates from the Men's Senior Baseball League in Austin had traveled to Phoenix to play in our age group's World Series. Teams from all over the world gathered every October in that city to play baseball on Major League's spring-training fields in an attempt to win a championship ring and recapture a bit of lost youth through our undying love for the game. I had been to the fall classic in the Valley of the Sun a few times and can hardly recall a greater joy. We played and watched baseball all day on big-time fields where the balls bounced true, and we slept like children each night, comforted to know that the next day would bring only fun and more baseball.

"If you would just go over to the lobby and have a seat, a nurse will call you back when they are ready for your pre-op."

Mary Lou and I did not talk. She knew I was afraid, not just of my loss of vision but also of an inability to maintain some semblance of a financial livelihood. She was worried, too, but, as always, remained strong and confident that our partnership could overcome any circumstances. Silence was more reassuring than analyzing our predicament; we would have to face the fact I had no idea what was coming next or how to resume earning an income. My consulting business had fallen off in the past year, and the distraction of an eye problem did not leave me the energy or concentration needed to pursue new clients or focus on business I had won. I kept trying, though without much success.

Mary Lou also understood how much I was missing baseball. As long as I could play, I was able to deceive myself slightly about my age and how I felt physically as the days rolled into years. Baseball requires two eyes, though, for depth of field; even in a senior league, the ball comes at you fast off an aluminum bat. Fly balls in the outfield are probably impossible to track with one eye, and it seemed foolish to even *think* about putting the barrel of the bat on a fastball.

Plus, it was silly to be thinking about baseball at all. I'd be 60 in a week, and Mary Lou and I had many other issues causing us to fret. Just prior to 9/11, we had built a new home in the Texas Hill Country, and I had left my job as an executive at a global public relations firm to start a private consulting practice. But the attack in New York wiped out my new business. When the world seems like it is on fire, not many companies or individuals worry about their public image. We were forced to live on credit cards and modest savings for more than a year, until I landed an anchor client. I also showed poor judgment after a former student intern asked me to start a video-technology company with him. I invested the remainder of my IRA and retirement but was forced from the company when I complained about bad strategic choices. After almost six years, there was no return on capital invested in the start-up, and Mary Lou and I were still struggling to pay our household bills.

And yet I dreamed of baseball as I sat in the hospital lobby. Although many of my teammates were former athletes still in their early 40s, I was faster than all but one of them. I took great pride in stealing bases and running down line drives that looked as if they were bound for a gap in the outfield and extra bases. There were some pitchers in our league, however, who still threw at around 80 mph, and, batting right-handed, I would be exposing my good left eye to a wild pitch simply for the joy of recreational baseball. That was probably an unwise risk if the other eye could not be preserved with surgery.

We were sitting and reading when Dr. D came through the lobby and stopped to say hello. Dangling his car keys loosely in his hand, he reminded me of a young tech executive who had just come in from driving his new BMW coupe through the Hill Country's twisting roads west of Austin.

"I have another case before yours," he said. "So I'll see you back there in a while. Shouldn't be too long."

"You think it's going to take this time?" I asked.

"We'll give you the best chance and the best care possible, Mr. Moore."

Dr. D was always circumspect; he consistently avoided being definitive, which is smart for any physician uncertain about a prognosis, but he also did not express confidence in his professional skills. Maybe doctors do not feel that is necessary, but patients want confident doctors. His communications were direct, but I thought they lacked an important degree of empathy. I often accused him of being too clinical, treating patients as cases instead of people. For a doctor, he also seemed incurious. I thought he might have been just as fulfilled screwing widgets into cars on an assembly line.

The morning of this particular surgery I was six weeks into what was to become a more-than-four-year struggle to save the vision in my right eye. My reappearance in the surgical theater would become so frequent that the anesthesiologist would ask, "You again? Like it here, do you?" My remaining financial resources were draining fast, but, as anyone who has had deteriorating eyesight will explain, there is nothing someone would not sacrifice to save one's natural ability to see the world. Our insurance policy under COBRA, in addition to high deductibles, only paid 70 percent of all costs. Consequently, each time I underwent an operation, either our debt increased or a bank account dwindled, often both.

As I lay in a hospital bed with an intravenous line, awaiting a sedative to calm me, I thought about the pre-operative diagnosis: a "recurrent retinal detachment of the right eye" and "proliferative vitreoretinopathy (PVR) of the right eye." This meant that, at some time, a hole or a tear had developed in my retina. Science still does not know exactly what causes those two things to happen, but they are likely the consequence of a thinner-than-normal area of the retina combined with vitreous traction that pulls at the retina until it tears. This may be driven by any number of genetic processes in the eye. Those holes or tears allow fluid to leak back behind the retina from the vitreous, which, combined with traction caused by the connected vitreous, create a rhegmatogenous detachment of the retina. Holes or tears do not always lead to detachments, however.

The diagnosis of PVR indicated that I had already crossed into a zone where my vision was never again going to return to previous levels of clarity. Dr. D, though, had not informed me of those details. I was undergoing a fibrotic, excessive wound healing caused by migrating and proliferating cells of the retinal pigmented epithelium (RPE), the cellular layer that provides nourishment to the neurosensory retina where light and movement are perceived. The transition of RPE cells into the vitreous and pre-retinal space allows them to proliferate and develop into membranes on the retina, which then cause contraction as they turn into a kind of scar tissue and prompt further detachment. Surgical repair has a moderate chance of success, but there is almost always a loss of associated vision.

My sense, as I was wheeled back to the operating room, was that I had asked sufficient questions of Dr. D over the course of multiple visits to his office. Short of studying biology and anatomy, however, there are always going to be issues a patient probably won't know. This, for me, was at the moral center of medicine. What is a doctor obligated to tell a patient? I had no idea that my case had been quickly complicated by PVR, and Dr. D never mentioned vitreous syneresis—a deterioration of the fibrous vitreous gel in the eye that turns it more into a liquid than a viscous substance. The more liquidity it acquires, the easier it leaks behind a hole or a tear and causes detachment. Syneresis is generally a breakdown of vitreous that occurs with aging.

Why was I not informed of these two developments?

The notion of "informed consent" seems to be limited by what a doctor feels is necessary to share. Is a patient informed if he or she signs a consent document that acknowledges there are risks with surgery? Those risks are listed only generally, like cardiac arrest or allergic reactions to drugs, not as dangers specific to certain procedures. Should an educated patient be given more information than an individual who might not exactly grasp the challenges of retinal detachment and vitreous syneresis? How much are we required to simply trust the skills of our physician? My auto mechanic always offered more detail than I was getting from the man who was about to put instruments into my eye.

Dr. D's surgical notes from that operation point out other topics to which I was oblivious before I gave what was considered informed consent. Although I was familiar with the use of scleral buckles, we'd never talked about taking that approach to resolving my detachment problem. Silicone buckles, or belts, sewn around the eye are almost quaint procedures given the technology presently available to retinal surgeons. Although they are still used, accomplished physicians increasingly consider the approach to be a blunt-force tactic in a practice like retinal surgery that often measures success in micrometers. There are far too many other sophisticated vitrectomy techniques that do not involve the trauma of externally pinching down the globe of the eye to force it to meet the detached retina or the risk of damaging the scleral wall or the muscles involved in eye movement.

Years after Dr. D placed the scleral buckle around my eye, I had a conversation with Steve Charles about the procedure. Charles had performed around 8,000 such operations in earlier years, but he judiciously avoids them now because there is a greater chance for a successful, uncomplicated outcome with vitrectomy techniques.

"There are several myths about how scleral buckles work," Charles told me. "What does it really do? It creates a shear zone plate. The conventional argument is that, if you bring the buckle halfway to the retina, it will 'settle.' But what about detachments in the top of the eye? When was the last time you saw something 'settle up?' You would not believe how many surgeons don't get what buckles do. Your job as a surgeon is to fix rhegmatogenous discontinuity. How do you do that? Do you smash the wall of the eye in with a scleral buckle? No, not really. The vitrectomy approach versus the scleral buckle approach is [as another ophthalmologist said] 'like using a bulldozer on the outside wall of a house instead of going inside and putting up wallpaper.'"

The question occurs, then, should Dr. D have told me he was using this relatively ineffective and nominally outdated technique? Or was I obligated to be a more informed patient and ask whether he had any intentions of employing a scleral buckle to fix my detachment? Regardless, while I was under anesthesia, he used Westcott scissors to cut a 360-degree conjunctival peritomy around the front of my eye, which gave him access to the four rectus muscles that moved the eye back and forth, up and down. (The conjunctiva is the tissue that lines the eyelids and the white surface of the eye and produces tears and protein for lubrication.)

"A 5-0 nylon suture was then placed in each of the four quadrants approximately 11–12 centimeters posterior to the limbus," Dr. D wrote in his postoperative notes. "The scleral buckle was then placed underneath the rectus muscles and through the sutures."

He then performed a sclerotomy, which is an incision in the sclera on the front of the eye "infero-temporally," or closest to the side of my head, and inserted a 23-gauge trocar through the cut and into the eye. The trocar, a tubelike cannula, was attached to an infusion line, which was to be used to flow fluid into my eye. Two other trocars were then put in the eye in spots on the opposite side of the cornea from the initial insertion.

The optical system Dr. D used to examine the retina was a BIOM, a wide-angle viewing system that does not contact the eye but provides a surgeon with an essential broad range of vision into the vitreous. Dr. D's notes said he used the BIOM to "assess the posterior pole," which meant he was looking directly at my optic nerve and the macula that provides central vision.

What he saw was disturbing: "a recurrent inferior detachment with a tear seen posterior to the previously placed laser." This meant that the laser I had received in Dr. D's office had held the targeted parts of the retina in place, but behind those spots, a new portion had torn loose. He used a vitrectomy probe—a high-speed cutter that is a part of the Constellation surgical platform designed by Steve Charles in conjunction with Alcon—and wrote afterward, "Additional vitreous was shaved to the vitreous base." Subsequently, Dr. D decided to infuse perfluoron (PFO) heavy liquid and position it over my optic nerve to sustain the reattachment of the retina. He referred to this in his notes by saying he chose to leave the perfluoron in place to "tamponade" the retina.

The language did not correctly describe the situation.

"The use of this word [tamponade] in retinal surgery is misleading," Charles told me later. "Tamponade means to plug, not press. Buoyancy will tell you where gas bubbles and heavy liquids go. PFO goes to the bottom. You keep the retina in place with gases and oils and heavy fluids by managing interfacial surface tension. You seal the break. Do it with gas or oil to keep it in place."

If the bottom of the retina is detached, Charles has developed a medium term PFO (heavy liquid) approach, but it must be removed in two weeks.

Dr. D removed the trocars from my eye after he saw that the retina was completely attached and tightened the scleral buckle to a "medium push" before tying the four 5-0 sutures. The scleral buckle was trimmed and placed under the four rectus muscles; he "re-approximated" the conjunctiva and sewed it back into position with 7-0 Vicryl sutures. A corticosteroid to manage inflammation and an antibiotic were injected into the sub-conjunctival space. My eye was patched, and I woke up in the recovery room.

"He said everything went great." Mary Lou was at my bedside as I regained consciousness.

"Uh, that's good."

My hand went to the large gauze patch that had been taped over my eye. There was complete blackness, something I had feared. Even as I was dealing with my grogginess after anesthesia, I was scared of losing the perception of light and movement in that eye. My mind was already making compromises: I would give up watching a baseball spin through the air. I just wanted the eye to function.

"Your retina is reattached now, Mr. Moore." Dr. D had moved through the curtains to my bedside. "I'll see you at the office tomorrow, and we can take off the patch."

"Am I going to see again?"

"We are doing everything possible to make that happen."

Again, I heard Dr. D's steady ambiguity, his unwillingness to connect to his patients' hopes. Maybe this was professionalism, an emotional detachment necessary for any physician who must inevitably confront failures at some point in their careers. My task to keep from becoming one of those failures was to go home and lie face down for a few weeks, to allow gas to float up to the back of my eye and to put pressure on the retina to hold it in position to heal.

Mary Lou drove home. I rolled down the truck's window and felt the dry October air rushing past on the highway. Autumn in Central Texas is the loveliest of all the seasons. Winds turn away from the Gulf's summer humidity and instead blow from the west across the Edwards Plateau and the Chihuahuan Desert. The air is comfortably warm, and the sky is a blue that is as pure as it must have been the day the world started spinning. People were running and cycling the trails around Town Lake, diving into the cold waters of Barton Springs, and sitting at cafés and beer joints on sun-drenched decks.

But all I felt was afraid.

SIX

Walkin' in Memphis

He drove his car to the iron gates and called up the hill to the big house on the security phone. Beautiful young women stood nearby, aimlessly talking and staring wistfully up the incline toward the mansion. A few of them asked if they could ride with him, just to get closer to the house, maybe to even catch a glimpse of Elvis Presley.

Steve Charles had to say no to their requests. The doctor had only been in town about a year in 1976, but his reputation was significant enough that the singer's half-brother, Billy Smith, had contacted Charles about problems with Elvis' eyes, which were frequently irritated by allergies. Elvis had a habit of using steroid drops to ease the itching and pain. The medication, however, often drove up the pressure inside his eyes, causing discomfort. Charles had brought with him a machine to measure intraocular pressure, but he was uncertain what to expect. He knew almost nothing about Elvis as a patient, though his medical-practice partner at the time claimed some doctor-patient relationship with the singer.

When the front door of the mansion opened, Charles was guided to a living room to wait. Linda Thompson, Elvis' girlfriend, a former beauty pageant queen, came in and introduced herself. She was wearing a white negligee.

"I'm sorry we don't have any alcohol to offer you," Thompson said. "We just have Coca-Cola."

"Oh, I'm fine. I don't drink."

"Let me go get Elvis."

A Memphis girl whose brother Sam was one of the singer's bodyguards, Thompson would later marry Olympic gold medalist decathlete Bruce Jenner and subsequently musician David Foster. She also became an accomplished lyricist and composer.

Elvis entered wearing a black Japanese kimono and immediately wanted to reward the doctor for making a house call to Graceland.

"He tried to give me a new Lincoln Continental limo," Charles recounted years later. "I couldn't take that. It was absurd. I told him I didn't need anything and that I had just come to check the pressure in his eyes. Although I didn't say it, I didn't even want an autograph or concert tickets."

Elvis, however, insisted on some form of remuneration for the doctor's services—even before they had been performed—and he brought out a Winchester 94, a Theodore Roosevelt commemorative issue known as a "saddle ring carbine." Charles had been home with his family, wearing blue jeans and an Oklahoma football jersey, when he got the call from Elvis' half-brother. He had simply put a white lab coat over his clothes before leaving for Graceland.

"And now, suddenly, I'm also holding a Chuck Connors–style *Rifleman* rifle over my shoulder, wearing jeans and a football jersey, and I'm standing there in Elvis' house. You can imagine how odd the whole thing felt to me, even before I had attended to his eyes."

The doctor did notice the singer's eyes, though. He appeared to be suffering from allergic conjunctivitis; the lining around his eyes was red and so swollen that it looked "like the tires on a Hummer," Charles recalled, possibly because of the singer's use of black dye on his otherwise gray-white eyebrows and hair. Charles suggested they travel to his office in order to conduct a more thorough exam.

"You mind if I take a shower before we go?" Elvis asked.

"Of course not."

Elvis and his girlfriend disappeared down the hall, but Charles could hear them singing the score of *The Sound of Music,* the film they had been watching when he arrived at Graceland. Presently, Elvis came back out dressed in blue tennis warm-ups. As they were leaving, Charles noticed that the King and his two bodyguards had .357 Magnum pistols stuffed into their waistbands.

"Do you drive fast?" Elvis asked Charles as they were leaving.

"Yes, I do."

"Okay, then we are taking my car."

The King apparently wanted to be safe.

Elvis had recently been criticized for youthful unrest during the early 1970s. A few reporters and commentators blamed his role in the birth of rock and roll for a rise in juvenile delinquency. The accusation rankled. On the drive to Charles' office, Elvis told the doctor how distressed he was about being misunderstood.

"I am not a rebel," the singer explained. "I'm a guy who was raised in Tupelo, Mississippi. I like music, especially the combination of gospel and R & B. Everybody's got me pegged wrong. I am very concerned about juvenile delinquency."

As they walked through the waiting room of Charles' office, Elvis noticed a *Sports Illustrated* with model Cheryl Tiegs on the cover. He stopped and pointed at her picture.

"You ever go out with her?" he asked Charles.

"Uh, no, I have not."

"Well, don't. She's dumb."

As Elvis took a seat in the exam chair, the singer kept talking about the law and his public image. He pulled out police badges from his wallet, which was thick with various forms of official identification.

"You know, I'm a deputy sheriff," Elvis said. "I'm a narc, too."

"Is this better? Or is this?" Charles interjected. He was refracting Elvis' eyesight, trying plus-three diopter lenses and then a minus three. "Which one is better?"

"Man, I don't know. You're the doc. You tell me."

By the time the exam had concluded, Elvis, the "narc," was insisting that Charles go with him on a drug bust. They drove to a troubled part of Memphis, and Elvis stopped the car next to what seemed to be a pool hall.

"The shades were pulled, and you couldn't really see inside," Charles remembered. "It was dark, and I told him we really didn't have any business there. He asked me to kick the tires on the car and reassured me we could convince anyone who came up that we were undercover. I said, 'You're an expert in rock and roll, and I'm an expert in eye surgery, but we are *not* undercover.'"

Elvis, of course, could not be undercover anywhere in the world.

Nevertheless, they got out of the car, and Charles kicked the tires as Elvis instructed in the kind of casual act that was supposed to offer a rationale for stopping. Eventually, people noticed the singer outside of the building and came out to greet the King of Rock and Roll, who was, improbably, in their neighborhood.

Narc or not, Chuck and Elvis returned to Graceland without making any arrests, and the singer invited Charles to hang around. He seemed lonely, Charles noted, even while surrounded by people.

The doctor spent the next two hours talking about the musician's favorite game of racquetball and getting a private tour of his famous home and collection of platinum and gold records. Elvis contacted Charles twice more to deal with his increased intraocular pressure and discomfort, but there was not enough time for them to develop a true personal connection.

And a year later, the King was gone.

CHOOSING TO BEGIN his professional life in Memphis had been mostly a serendipitous development. After training physicians from around the world during his two years at the National Eye Institute, Charles understood the value of being centrally located in the United States. At a few conferences, he had encountered a Memphis retinal surgeon who invited him to join an established practice. The business relationship ultimately failed and was quite financially costly for Charles, but he had found a home in Memphis, where he later established his own practice, the Charles Retina Institute.

Even as he dealt with the difficult repercussions—financial and otherwise—of the failed practice partnership, Charles saw hundreds of patients. His skills had not been diminished. In fact, the doctor made important new clinical observations and gathered data on two conditions related to the retina that had previously not been noticed or recorded. Both became critical in follow-up care for retina patients.

Charles had learned from Robert Machemer that proliferation, the development of membranes, excessive and recurrent tissue healing problems on the retina, was mostly prevented by the removal of all the vitreous inside the eye. While treating patients in Memphis, though, Charles noted that was not really the case. Even with the complete removal of all epiretinal membranes (ERMs—growth of contractile scar tissue on the retina), which accumulated upon the retinal surface of some patients after surgery, proliferation of membrane tissue still recurred in a significant number of patients. This happened even after the retina had been treated with scissors segmentation, a technique developed by Charles for diabetic traction retinal detachments. He had also designed a technique using forceps to peel less adherent epimacular membranes (similar tissue growth on the surface of the macula), as well as membranes caused by proliferative vitreo retinopathy (PVR), and it became a widely adopted technique.

The level of precision required to operate on the human retina is largely incomprehensible to the average person. When Charles looked at diabetic retinas with traction, retinal detachment with highly adherent ERMs, he believed that they could not be safely removed. It occurred to him that by cutting them into sections with micro scissors, he would reduce the tangential pulling force on the retina. The objective was to divide the ERM into sites with the most vascularized adherence to the retina and then deal separately with each of those tissue "epicenters."

Initially, Charles used vertical scissors in the eye and placed one blade between the retina and the membrane; the other was above the surface of the ERM. As the segments were cut and separated from each other, the force caused by traction on the retina was reduced and even eliminated. The reason for such segmentation, in most cases, is that the ERM is too adherent to the eye to peel. Eventually, Charles began cutting ERMs with curved scissors; that reduced the risk of retinal puncture and made it considerably easier to get between the ERM and the retina. In some cases, though, residual tissue remained on the retina even after segmentation, which prompted the doctor to develop scissors delamination, a procedure to cut the membrane off instead of cutting it up.

Because retinal tissue is delicate and thin, it is very fragile. Any surgical approaches must be precise. When Charles began segmentation of membranes lying over the retina, it enabled reattachment. His procedures had an immediate positive impact on the vision of diabetic patients losing sight. Using scissors segmentation to manage traction retinal detachment meant more people with diabetes who had previously been losing their vision would instead be able to continue seeing.

ERMs in diabetic retinas often resulted in small areas of chronic retinal elevation that could cause retinal holes and rhegmatogenous retinal detachments. But two years after he had developed segmentation, Dr. Charles designed and successfully executed a new technique called scissors delamination, which enabled removal of most, if not all, the membranes. First, segmentation cut up the ERM; second delamination cut it off. Using curved scissors once again to reduce the risk of impaling the retina, Charles inserted the open blades under the edge of the ERM, felt for an attachment point, and cut. Pulling back slightly, he opened the blades a little and felt for another attachment to cut. Because ERMs are taut, they scroll up for easy grasping and removal from the retinal surface. Increasingly, Charles performed segmentation and delamination in a single operation.

The doctor had other things on his mind beside surgery. Charles was an active father, participating in the raising of his daughters—he now had three—and settling into a new home despite working long hours. These were not casual responsibilities. Throughout his life and career, Charles has made it clear that nothing is more important than being a father and, eventually, a grandfather, and he has been unfailingly devoted to his daughters.

Yet his focus on improving surgical outcomes never wavered.

In his first year in Memphis, Charles noticed another dynamic in the retina that called for treatment to prevent visual loss. The clinical concept became known as anterior loop traction. During surgery for retinal detachments from PVR, the doctor observed that radial collagen fibers previously in contact with the retina were contracting and pulling the equatorial retina forward. These were the sheets of tissue extending from the retinal equator at the back edge of the vitreous base toward the pars plana, and they were contracting as a result of a hypocellular process caused by retinal pigment epithelial, or glial cells. The shortening of the fibers pulled the equatorial retina forward and also created a circumferential fold. Charles reported that shearing the fibers with the vitreous cutter or scissors released the retina and made it possible to achieve reattachment.

After Charles arrived in Memphis in 1975, his mechanical and electrical engineering efforts, coupled with clinical observation, led to an astonishing list of innovations that have had a cumulative impact on retinal treatment and have also become the standard of care for the subspecialty. Whenever he encountered a challenge in treatment that might be improved by a better or completely new tool, the doctor either redesigned one or created something previously unseen. The goal was always to reduce risk and improve outcomes. The list of Charles innovations, even just those that came in the first five years of his practice in Memphis, is astonishing when considered in the context of a doctor with a burgeoning patient load, three daughters, and a practice to help manage.

Charles' developments spawned techniques that are still utilized as the standard of care after more than four decades. These include forceps membrane peeling, air-silicone exchange, scissors segmentation and delamination of ERMs, retinectomy, punch-through retinotomy for the removal of subretinal bands, aspirating pars plana lensectomy, endophotocoagulation, flute cannula, linear suction, suction-only modality of the foot pedal, subretinal scissors, MicroVit proportional scissors, subretinal forceps, illuminated intraocular foreign-body forceps, MicroVit Vitrectomy System, volumetric power gas injector, infusion sleeve for the vitreous cutter, bipolar bimanual intraocular diathermy clips, irrigating fundus contact lens with integrated handle, filter for fluorescein angioscopy during vitrectomy, and endophotocoagulation adapter for Clinitex Log III portable xenon. The doctor also added three more clinical concepts to his observations: the proliferative vitreoretinopathy effect of a silicone-gas retinal interface; the compartmentalization, or barrier concept; and anterior hyaloidal fibrovascular proliferation, also called retrolenticular neovascularization.

Any one of these advancements is worthy of acclaim and perhaps more than any other physician and researcher might accomplish in a career. Taken as a whole, they have moved an entire profession in the direction of greater achievement for the care of people with retinal problems. No one believes that more than his colleagues. Julia Haller, M.D., who serves as Ophthalmologist-in-Chief at Wills Eye Hospital, the oldest and largest eye hospital in the U.S., is convinced retinal surgery would have taken considerably longer to evolve without her friend Steve Charles.

"There was a kind of a critical mass, a coming together in retina," she said. "It was almost an explosive time because so much of how we do modern surgery was developed in those years, and Steve was right there at the forefront pushing the process and developing instruments, using his engineering brain with his surgeon's insights. We would have been at a much different place without him. He's just been such a critical innovator and leader and has really driven the evolution in our field."

Charles' advancements were elemental to improving care and

outcomes. The devices, however, were individual hand tools and required significant surgical skill to learn. Differing functionalities meant that various instruments were inserted into the eye and then removed through the single, penetrating incision in the sclera. Vitreous could be cut and removed through that single opening, but it was difficult to get enough light to see the interior of the eye, and cutters were unable to effectively accomplish every procedure. These challenges began to drive change.

Only a few years after Charles' arrival in Memphis, a salesman approached the doctor with a system that he said could improve vitreoretinal surgery. The doctor had already heard of a new methodology for vitrectomy using three separate smaller openings into the eye, which allowed for more physician flexibility and capabilities in the intraocular space. The technique and technology had been developed by Dr. Conor O'Malley and engineer Ralph Heinz. The procedure used a 20-gauge hollow pipe for inserting tools, considerably smaller than the 16-gauge hollow needle deployed in Machemer's VISC. O'Malley and Heinz had designed an operating platform called the Ocutome 800. It included a lightweight, bellows-driven, reusable axial cutter. Instead of a syringe to aspirate fluid and vitreous from the eye, the Ocutome used foot-pedal-controlled aspiration that was managed by the surgeon using an on-and-off foot pedal.

O'Malley, who came from an Irish family of 35 physicians, realized that multiple small incisions were far less traumatic to the eye than a larger, single sclerotomy. That approach enabled surgical flexibility, as well as always-on infusion for more accurately controlling air and fluid pressures. The Ocutome 800, which was patented in 1972 and sold by Berkeley Bioengineering, had a separate cannula to introduce saline into the eye for maintaining intraocular pressure. The other two lines enabled doctors to deploy endo-illumination and the vitreous cutter. The cutter could be removed for the introduction of a laser probe and other tools, such as scissors and forceps, while the other hand positioned the endo-illuminator, and the saline infusion line maintained normal pressure. O'Malley's reduction in the tool gauge size from 16 to 20 also made possible much smaller incisions.

O'Malley was onto something big. His notion of three small incisions instead of a single, large sclerotomy led to a trend that has guided surgical approaches for virtually all types of operations and increased positive results using a minimally invasive tactic. Recovery tends to be accelerated when trauma is reduced, but the Ocutome also increased doctors' capabilities and expanded the types of retinal problems that could be treated.

O'Malley, although by nature a private and introverted man, was aware of the importance of his platform and techniques. He took the same approach to advancement as Robert Machemer did when he was promoting vitrectomy in a closed intraocular space. O'Malley and Charles conducted workshops around the country for doctors interested in the Ocutome and the three-port vitrectomy. He also published numerous articles so surgeons could understand the use of his patented system of instruments and their new techniques. The three-port vitrectomy became the standard of care in the vitreoretinal subspecialty of ophthalmology.

"Machemer's VISC was conceptually sound, but nobody used it much because it was big and clunky," said medical historian Kirk Packo. "O'Malley's Ocutome was wonderful and useful, and it spread through the profession like the computer. It really took off."

Charles played a significant role in the proliferation of the Ocutome 800 through medical circles. During the first year, only a handful of the machines were sold, but after Charles began using it and speaking about its advantages at professional conferences, the

Ocutome sold around 500 in its second year. When Charles spoke at a demonstration of the Ocutome 800 at the annual American Academy of Ophthalmology's meeting for vitreo-retinal surgeons, the room quickly filled, and there were lines to get information. Doctors were soon acquiring the platform at a rate of 75 per month.

Though the Ocutome was a major improvement for retinal surgery, the machine was still imperfect. Its vitreous cutter was non-disposable and constantly needed repairs and rehoning that required a return to the manufacturer. Surgeons learned to keep at least three vitreous cutters on a nearby tray, because blades dulled quickly, and they often failed to function. Illumination offered by the Ocutome was less than optimal, and the aspiration process, now foot controlled, needed improvements in speed and proportional control.

What O'Malley had done, however, was start ripples that would build into a wave of transformation. Charles envisioned even greater potential for the Berkeley Bioengineering Ocutome 800. He began to think about adapting his new techniques—like internal drainage of subretinal fluid and endophotocoagulation, among others—to a system with greater capabilities. Very quickly, he became convinced there would be broad adoption of such a platform and that vitreoretinal surgery could be made dramatically more effective. To the surprise of no one who knew him, he immediately got to work on engineering a machine to provide even greater improvement to eye care.

SEVEN

The *Texas Eagle*

There were two other patients wearing eye patches in Dr. D's waiting room the morning after my surgery. They seemed almost cheery, and both were considerably younger than me. Neither looked weary from their first night of living facedown while waiting for the gas in their eye to help the retina heal. One, a woman in her 20s, had her legs crossed and was bouncing her draped foot energetically. She flipped through a copy of *Cosmopolitan,* which I hoped she had brought with her and did not pick up off a table in my retinal surgeon's lobby. The other person was a middle-aged man chatting softly with his wife. Neither of them seemed too distracted by the gauze and tape on their faces.

I, however, was anxious. I had almost wanted to tear off the eye cover in the middle of the night to see if I might have vision through the gas he'd used to help keep the retina attached. The buckle encircling my eye was a permanent fixture that was supposed to have changed eye shape and reduce traction. Of course, I had been told not to expect to see until my body began to absorb the gas and the bubble shrank. Dr. D had said that my first sight would be like I was coming up from underwater and looking above the waterline.

While this seemed a perfectly reasonable description, I also found it a bit unsettling, considering that drowning was included in that imagery. Nevertheless, I forgave Dr. D. I figured he was a better surgeon than poet; at least, I hoped that to be the case.

I was dealing with something else physical that I could not name. Every time I confronted my eye problem and thought of blindness, a wave of nausea caused contractions in my stomach and my bowels. Never before in my life had I felt so completely helpless and unprepared. Suddenly, nothing was in my control. There was no exercise to perform, no medicine to take, no prescribed diet. Even if I had endless financial resources, they would be of no value against sour luck and bad biology. The apparent futility of my situation had prompted me to lean against the wall outside Dr. D's office and empty my breakfast onto the ground, a session of vomiting that ended with dry heaves and a burning throat before I was able to regain composure and enter the doctor's lobby for my postoperative examination.

I was trying to figure out what type of assessment Dr. D could make on my eye if I could not see out through the gas. Wouldn't it be impossible for him to look into my eye *through* the gas and determine if the retina were holding in place? Suddenly, it was time for my examination.

"Did you sleep okay, Mr. Moore?" Dr. D passed a light in front of the eye, but I barely perceived its presence.

"The drugs helped," I said. "But it was kind of hard with my face buried in a pillow or my head hanging off the side of the bed."

"You'll have the desk today, and the collar for your bed?"

"Yes, we were told they'd arrive today."

"Very good. As you know, it is critical to keep your head down."

"Doctor, no one is more determined in this than me. My wife

drove me here while I stared at the floorboards. I can assure you I will not see the sky for a few weeks."

My neck was hurting, and it felt good when Dr. D asked me to look up as he pressed an ultrasound wand across my closed eyelid.

"The gas is where it needs to be, and from what I can tell with the ultrasound and visual exam, the retina appears attached," Dr. D said. "We can't be completely certain, but things look good."

"So how long before I can see again?"

"We have four to six weeks before your body completely absorbs the gas, but in about half that time you should begin to see around the bubble, assuming the retina has remained attached."

"Is there any reason to think it won't?"

"No, but we always have to be cautious." Dr. D had his back to me and was punching information into my file on the computer. "I put in an appropriate amount of laser, drained the subretinal fluid, and the gas is also holding it in place for complete reattachment."

I considered laser to be much like welding, which was probably another bad analogy. The heat from the laser created spots on the retina, which were, essentially, locations where the heat coagulated tissue and scarring developed after the burn. Retinal tissue healing created a seal around the first tear to keep fluid from leaking and causing a recurrent tear or, worse, a detachment.

The next two weeks were horrible. A mad scientist's version of a third-grader's desk was set up and located not far from the television. My downward-tilted cranium rested in a padded notch that was aligned with a double mirror, which allowed me to see the screen of my laptop or the TV without image reversal. Working the keyboard was nearly impossible and required my arms to be extended until they dropped in pain and exhaustion. When I grew weary, I took a sleep aid, slid the horseshoe collar between the mattress and box spring on our bed so that the padded loop protruded to act as a head support, and lay face down, as though I were preparing for a massage.

I was not unaccustomed to personal discipline and was confident I could handle this constant looking down to save my eyesight. My determination had been sharpened through years of distance running, getting up early each morning and knocking off 10-mile runs to train for competitive races. I could lower my head and stare at ants for weeks on end if it meant that my eye would regain some useful vision. I did not know how difficult it might be to accomplish my writing or complete projects for consulting clients, but nothing was more valuable than eyesight. I assumed I would find a way to sustain my business and my writing and also reacquire a clear eye.

I simply was unable to find a comfortable manner, though, in which to position my hands and arms over the keys of my laptop. Writing continued to be slowed by cramps and having to constantly refocus my healthy left eye. My brain was learning to process data from one eye instead of two, and it was almost impossible to read at a normal pace. Headaches came fast, a malady I had never experienced other than after too many glasses of wine over dinner. When a consulting client called for advice or insights, their concerns seemed trivial compared to my circumstances. I tried not to be too curt, but I kept thinking about the three holes that had been poked into my eye for the pars plana vitrectomy and the injection of gas after the laser to seal the leaks around the original tear in my retina.

A little over a week after the surgery, when I was still dreaming about how soon I could look back up, my sister called to say that my mother was going into hospice and did not have much time.

"I can't fly, Bev," I explained. "I had retinal detachment surgery, and there's gas in my eye."

"Does something happen if you fly?"

"Uh, yeah. The gas expands, which is not a good thing."

"Oh, I guess not."

I almost laughed at the image of my eye exploding all over my seatmate's laptop keyboard on a crowded flight: *Oh, I'm sorry. Let me hit the flight-attendant call button. Oops! There's a part of my iris on your shift key, dude.*

"I guess I'll have to take the train, Bev."

"How long of a train ride is it from Austin to Lansing?"

"Probably a long one."

"I know she wants to see you. She keeps talking about you all the time."

"Well, I won't be able to leave for several more days because of this gas in my eye, but I will get a ticket and head up. After I end this head-down stuff."

"Very funny, little brother."

Almost three weeks passed before I was unafraid of lifting my head and getting on a train. My main concern was that I had no sense that the bubble was shrinking, because I still saw nothing. Even more worrisome, I had to go back to Dr. D because my right eye had begun to wander, a condition known as strabismus. Blindness, a term I hesitated to use because of its finality, had affected the rectus muscles that controlled movement in my right eye. The muscles were, essentially, nonresponsive. I was given a patch and told to wear it to rest the eye, and movement would return to normal in a week or two. I strapped the patch on and looked into the mirror with a bit of trepidation. The effect was both disconcerting and intriguing.

Boarding the Amtrak train in Austin wearing an eye patch, I felt a bit like a John le Carré character trying to avoid being caught on an airplane. My laptop and mobile phone kept me connected to the real world, however, and disabused me of any romantic self-deceptions. My mother was making her exit, and I needed to be in Michigan, though her transfer to hospice from her assisted-living residence had been postponed by her improved health. Ma was always a hypochondriac and had fretted over her well-being since having a colostomy operation in her early 40s. After the surgery, Ma never saw herself as a whole person again. She often called 911 for headaches, and though she was in her early 80s, she suspected every twinge marked the onset of a heart attack. There were times she would call 911, vacuum my sister's house while waiting for EMTs to show up, and lie on the couch when finished until the ambulance arrived to take her to the emergency room.

My love of train travel was sorely tested on the northbound trip. The *Texas Eagle* took 11 hours to reach Texarkana, a distance covered by car on Interstates 30 and 35 in about half of that time. Passenger cars on the train were generally clean, uncrowded, and comfortable, though, and there was so much room in the reclining seats I felt no need to buy a berth, which was, in any case, absurdly expensive. When the train turned north up the Mississippi River Valley, passing rich bottomlands on the way to St. Louis and Chicago, I sat under the overhead light, reading with one eye and watching fellow travelers sneak sidelong glances at my eye patch as they walked up the aisle. From time to time I turned my reduced gaze on the passing landscape.

Lights from the farmhouses went on in the distance as I rose to make my way to the dining car near the front of the train. Limited seating meant that travelers were required to eat with strangers. Oddly, when I arrived, there was an empty booth, and because I was not feeling social, I slipped into it. A white-jacketed waiter arrived almost immediately, and I ordered a glass of Cabernet. As he stepped away, I looked at my phone to read a news story.

"May I?"

I looked up at a well-dressed woman in her early 40s. She was blonde and expensively attired in a long black skirt and loose blouse, with large chunky jewelry.

"Yes, certainly. Please." I motioned for her to sit.

We exchanged cordialities, and the waiter arrived to take her drink order. As we both sipped wine and scanned the limited menu, I assumed there would be no conversation, but we began chatting comfortably. After I had explained why my wife and daughter had been unable to join me on the trip, the woman took her right hand off her lap to slowly brush hair away from her face. She wanted to make certain I saw the outsize diamond that undoubtedly cost more than my house. Such an overdone adornment has always prompted me to make generalizations about the woman who is wearing it. But the ground rules had been firmly established for us, and we conversed easily.

"I started out with a good chance at a fulfilled career," she told me. "I finished law school and was with a small firm in Effingham, Illinois, and then, I fell in love and got married."

"Kids and all that?"

"Yes, two, very early. They're grown now. Of course, I had two more marriages before I stopped hating myself for giving up my future."

"Amazing the decisions that we're forced to make when we are young, eh?"

"I suppose." She paused and offered a wan smile at the waiter when he brought our dinners. We both began to eat.

"Quite nice," I said. "Not what I expected on a train."

"No." She looked at me. "May I ask you a sort of personal question?"

She did not seem to be a person who had any real interest in my personal life. I immediately assumed she was going to ask me about the patch over my eye. I wondered how people could comfortably inquire about a condition that was apparent from the patch. Whose business was it, other than the wearer's?

"I don't mind, I suppose."

"I was wondering how you lost your eye and what you went through to adjust. My nephew had an accident very young, and he never quite adjusted to only having one eye."

The question, though expected, felt to me more personal than if she had inquired about my sex life. Since the issue had arisen with my retina, I'd been inclined to make light of the situation. Now, I had a couple of glasses of wine in my belly, and I wanted a laugh.

"Well, I work for one of those international security companies," I said.

"What does that mean?"

"We help businesses keep their interests safe around the world."

"With guns?"

"We try to avoid that. Things get complicated." I had lowered my voice slightly conspiratorially.

"Oh, I see." She was finishing her third glass of Pinot Grigio. "Did you get injured?"

"Yes, I am afraid I had the bad fortune of being on a freighter off the coast of Africa when pirates tried to board."

"Oh, my." She leaned forward. "What happened?"

I could not go on. I started to laugh.

"Oh, God, I was going to tell you that one of the pirates and I got into a fight, and he sliced my eye with a knife. But I couldn't keep a straight face.

"I've got a detached retina," I continued. "It's problematic, but I am hoping it will heal and my vision will be back to normal."

"Oh," she said, not quite openly offended by my fantasy exploits.

"People seem to want a romantic or adventurous story to go with an eye patch," I said.

"Yes, it would seem so." She looked out the window at the flickering lights dotting the farmland. "I think I'm going to skip my coffee and call it a night. Do enjoy your trip."

I wondered if she might have believed me had I told her I was taking a train from Texas to Michigan for a last visit with my mother. Or that I could not fly because there was gas in my eye, and it could rupture under expansion in a low-pressure airplane cabin. Then, I realized I did not care. I had almost been entertained.

As I drove a rental car from the Lansing train station to the village where my mother was living, I removed the patch. I wanted to see if my eye were back in its proper position and moving in unison with the healthy one. I decided to not wear the covering when I was with Ma; she did not need additional worries. She had always been adept at manufacturing crises, even though circumstance and poor choices had provided her with more than a sufficient inventory of challenges and disappointments.

Ma was sitting in the living room when I arrived and did not recognize me. I did not get her attention until I was almost at her side. Her face was pale and soft and suggested she was not pleased with how she was living. My mother's life was, in fact, as amazing as it was tragic. During World War II, she had fallen in love with an American soldier who was shipping out from her hometown of St. John's, Newfoundland. Pregnant before he departed, she found herself a 17-year-old mother on a train to the southern United States en route to live with in-laws she had never met. She would remain there until her husband returned from Europe.

Nothing went right. She lived in a sharecropper's shack in the middle of a vast cotton patch with her indifferent and disaffected in-laws and waited for my father to return and lead her to a better life. But when he got back to Mississippi, Daddy only chopped cotton and tried to save enough for a piece of land of his own. Five years passed before they left on a bus for Michigan in search of more rewarding work. Ma had an eighth-grade education, and Daddy had quit school at age 16 during the Great Depression to work in the fields. Their prospects were not good.

Ma became a waitress in burger joints, and Daddy got a job as a laborer in a car plant. Six kids, a $10,000 mortgage they could not afford, 60-to-80-hour workweeks, and my father's psychological frailty led to violence, domestic abuse, and mental breakdowns. The police came to our house often, and Daddy was finally institutionalized, enduring more than 20 electroshock therapy treatments. Ma finally divorced him after 21 years of marriage, but she no longer expected happiness or any type of fulfillment. Her children struggled to reject her sadness and seek their own lives of accomplishment and joy. We knew she loved us, but we could not understand her surrender to melancholy when she was only in her 40s.

I remembered the first time I had said good-bye to Ma. At 17, after finishing high school, I had wanted to see America. I had a backpack and a pocketful of one- and five- dollar bills. My mother, who had always smelled of fried food from the restaurants where she worked, held me tightly, trying to convince me there was no need to leave. She might have forbidden me to hitchhike west, but she probably knew I would not listen. My sweet mother had come to America for love and money and had ended with a job that provided her with nickel-and-dime tips from truckers and factory workers. Now, even her finest possessions, her children, were beginning to leave.

This last good-bye was going to be more painful.

I finally stopped thinking about my eye and turned my attention to the woman whose sundered life had given me chances. Slowly, she recognized me and tried to stand to offer a hug, but I leaned over and kept her seated.

A woman with papery skin and a frail neck walked up to me as I took my seat. She had been taking tiny steps around the room.

"I just came here to see if I could get someone to help me," she said. "Can you help me?"

"I would if I knew how," I answered. "But I don't."

The woman turned and teetered in a new direction, like one of those robot vacuum cleaners that has just bumped into a wall.

Ma stared at the front door of the assisted-living home, and I reached over and touched her hair to make certain she knew I was still at her side. She had colored her hair for many years but had let it go completely gray as she grew more sedentary.

"Son?" She touched my forearm. "Did you come up here from Texas just to see me?"

"Of course, Ma. I'll always be coming back home to you. You know that. I told you that the first time I took off with my backpack, remember?"

"Yep. I do. Would you help me now?" She was still looking at the door and had not turned in my direction.

I was starting to think that Ma thought her youth and health were on the other side of the door of that home. In her mind, it seemed, she continued to come and go as she wished, but her body was obviously failing.

"What do you need, Ma?"

"Son, I need you to get me out that door and down to the Canadian border. If you can just get me out that door and down to that big bridge in Detroit, I'll be okay. I can get across."

"Ma, you can't travel by yourself. You know that."

"Don't you tell me, son."

"Where would you go when you got across the bridge?"

"Home. I'd go home. To St. John's. And I'd never leave again. I should've listened to my mother and never left with your dad."

"You made a pretty good go of things for a girl a long way from home, Ma."

"No, I didn't."

"Well, what if I got you across that bridge to Canada? Then what? I have to get back to Texas and work."

"I'll just use this walker, and I'll walk and walk and walk until I flop over tired. Then, I'll sleep right there and start the next day and keep doing that until I get to St. John's."

"It's a long way to walk to Newfoundland, Ma, and you've got to get on board a ship, too, remember? Besides, if you got there, who would take care of you? Les and Brian and Gertie are gone now."

"What do you mean who will take care of me?" She raised her whispery voice. "I'll take care of me. I always have, haven't I?"

"But, Ma, you're . . ."

"You don't tell me anything, son, you hear? I'll get me a job at one of those restaurants down on the harbor, and I'll rent me a room off Water Street. I just need you to get me to the border, and then you can go on to Texas. Don't you worry about how I'll get home. You never let me worry about you."

"I know, Ma. But you did, anyway. I'm sorry."

I did not tell her about my eye. She would have spent the rest of her short time obsessing over my healthy one and the prospects it might also develop a problem.

And it already felt like a season of loss. A wet October wind was stripping the bright leaves off of maple trees beside the house where Ma lived. I knew that I would never be with her again, but I felt a need to get home to Texas and ask Dr. D why none of my vision had returned.

"I love you, Ma," I said. "But I have to go now."

"I know, son. I love you too. I wish I could go too."

I hugged her, and as I went out the door, I could feel her gaze following me. In the car, I pulled the eye patch out of my bag, slipped the band around my head, and draped the cloth over my eye. I waited a moment to adjust to the feeling and drove into the rising wind toward the train station and home.

I cried most of the drive.

EIGHT

A Man and His Machines

A gun to the head was no way to treat an honored guest. Steve Charles was afraid to move. The doctor stared straight ahead at the podium where he would soon be speaking about one of history's great scientists. He was having trouble processing the idea that in this prestigious auditorium he was being forced to confront gunmen.

"Don't move," a voice said. "Don't even twitch."

The metal was cold against his skin, and Charles felt a second barrel press against the other side of his neck.

"I . . . I don't understand," he said.

"Do not turn around."

"Believe me, I won't. But I'm not a threat to anyone. I'm a speaker here to honor the late Dr. Michaelson. Please don't . . ."

"Doesn't matter who you are. Our job is to protect the prime minister. Just don't do anything that makes us think you aren't a speaker or a scientist or a doctor or whatever you are."

"I can assure you, I won't."

The voice went silent as the chilly metal was pulled away from the doctor's head. He did not turn around to see who had threatened him, and in less than a minute, Israeli Prime Minister Yitzhak Shamir took his seat in front of Charles.

The doctor was in Jerusalem at a medical conference in 1984 to give a speech honoring the legacy of Israeli researcher Isaac Michaelson, a man whose work, like that of Charles, had an incalculable impact on the prevention of blindness. Michaelson had theorized that vascularization in the human body did not happen without a natural biological stimulus, a kind of trigger, which he called "Factor X." Michaelson believed Factor X was a peptide that signaled the body when it needed to increase the oxygen supply to certain parts of the anatomy, and that prompted the growth of blood vessels. Three decades later, his findings led to the development of a drug to prevent neovascularization in the eye, which finally made treatable the previously blinding disease of wet age-related macular degeneration (wAMD) through a series of injections.

Instead of talking about medicine and research during the conference, however, Charles kept getting pulled into side conversations about God and morality and how that needed to inform a physician's work. The guns, fortunately merely an annoyance, were an additional distraction.

"Early on in the conference, I was talking to one of my colleagues," Charles said. "He was a leader at one of our most prestigious med schools in the U.S. And he just kept talking about how much Judeo-Christian history we all needed to study and know, have faith, be spiritual. I wasn't interested in any of that. I care about making blind people see, and I didn't care about religion. So, when I get asked if there is a God, I say that's unknowable. And it doesn't matter, because it doesn't reduce the majesty of the hummingbird or the Grand Canyon."

Charles drifted away from the conference, missing the remainder of the agenda, because he was becoming intrigued by a new idea. The concept began to consume his mind, and the doctor eventually entered what he later described as a fugue state. Charles had no way of knowing what was happening to him as imagery and plans raced through his brain. All his training in medicine and mechanical and electrical engineering appeared to be converging into a single idea.

"In retrospect, everything felt like it happened without my conscious choosing," Charles said, decades removed from the experience. "This wasn't anything I had planned or had been dreaming about, but when it began to take shape, I realized it was a critical advancement, and it was sort of materializing in front of me and in my mind on a couple of different levels."

After asking the hotel's concierge for poster boards and markers, Charles spent the next three days forgoing meals and sleep and designing a device that would be known as the Ocular Connection Machine (OCM). He was on the verge of making another breakthrough in the way microsurgery was performed on the human eye. Charles wanted to drive the functionality of an operating platform with fluidics and to manage the system using fluidic circuit boards. In his hotel room, he also wrote out the core modules needed for a xenon light source, dual-actuation disposable vitreous cutters, and power-driven scissors and forceps.

The OCM seemed like it might become the second evolutionary step in vitreoretinal surgery almost a decade after Conor O'Malley's Ocutome 800. For years, Charles, who had widely promoted the Ocutome and had significant responsibility for its success, had looked very closely at that platform's functionality and how it might be advanced.

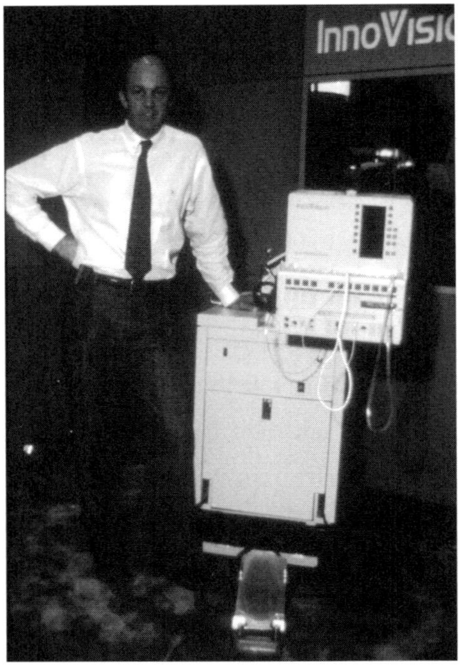

Charles and his first surgical platform: Ocular Connection Machine

The most critical issue with the Ocutome 800 system was the vitreous cutter, which wore out after about seven or eight uses and had to be returned to the factory for sharpening. The Ocutome cutter was considerably lighter than Machemer's VISC, and, instead of using a rotary action, which often caused vitreous to wrap around the inner needle and create intraocular traction, it employed a guillotine cutting process. Unfortunately, the tool, only 22 grams in weight, was in consistent need of repair and sharpening. Charles' goal with the OCM would be to improve cutting efficiency and longevity of the key instruments on his platform.

Before he developed the OCM, however, Charles began to apply most of his innovative techniques for vitreoretinal surgery to the Ocutome 800, which had been acquired by Coopervision after the sale of Berkeley Bioengineering. Working with Carl Wang and his engineering team, who had also moved to Coopervision after the Berkeley purchase, Charles began a collaboration that incorporated his personal surgical advancements into a platform, called the Ocutome 8000, which significantly transcended the performance of the earlier technology. Surgeons would be able to perform internal drainage of subretinal fluid through the vitreous cutter, use forceps for membrane peeling, segment and delaminate membranes on the retina with specially designed scissors, and execute fluid-air exchange along with endophotocoagulation.

Perhaps even more importantly for patients, the Ocutome 8000 system employed linear suction to remove vitreous, hemorrhage, scar tissue, and liquids from the eye. The flow of that substance was controlled by a proportional foot pedal, which brought nuance to a process that had previously been a preset vacuum managed only by an on-and-off foot switch. Charles and Wang advanced aspiration with proportional control on the Ocutome 8000. Linear suction and the alteration of the cutting process from rotary to guillotine reduced chances of complications during surgery and improved the odds of successful outcomes.

The Ocutome 8000 laid a foundation for numerous other technological improvements in vitreoretinal surgery. Dr. Brooks McEwen, for example, developed an air pump to sustain intraocular pressure, which replaced a syringe for fluid-air exchange inside of the eye. Fluid air exchange technique was engineered by Charles to avoid having a needle in a deflated eye after fluids had been removed, the technique used by Robert Machemer. The fluid-air exchange avoided deflating the eye, because air was injected while fluid was aspirated, thereby maintaining normal pressure in the eye. McEwen took this a step further by providing a continuous air source to replace the syringe.

Getting useful tamponade substances into the eye was improved when Charles and Wang invented power-gas and power-silicone oil injectors. (Tamponade, as a descriptive, is often misused in retinal surgery. Oil and gas inside of the eye are used because of a surface-tension effect, not pressure.) The linear suction Charles and Wang invented and added to the Ocutome 8000 has been used consistently since its launch on every phaco-emulsification and vitrectomy machine. There was also an integrated light source and an ultrasonic fragmenter to remove lens material.

The impulse to view the Ocutome 8000 as just a machine for surgery tends to overlook its importance in the evolution of eye care. Steve Charles and other physician innovators in the retina field were simply developing handheld tools driven by various power sources and fluidics. By bringing diverse functionalities together into the single OCM system, thinking was altered. Charles began to contemplate a platform, simple to use, which employed all his latest techniques and technology. The impact of this idea, if properly executed by design, was likely to result in improved chances for saving eyesight and considerably more efficiency in the operating room.

There was probably no time in his career where the confluence of Steve Charles' engineering and medical skills had a greater influence on the direction of vitreoretinal surgery. A doctor thinking like an engineer to solve biological problems with mechanical insights was a rarity in any type of medicine. The fact that Charles was performing in a profession that was, essentially, microsurgery, meant his ideas had a greater chance of making a difference, because technology was needed to go beyond the skills of the human hand and eye.

Michael Papac, Ph.D., a manager of engineering at medical device manufacturer Alcon, worked with Charles in the design and creation of advanced surgical platforms. Papac believes Charles' perspective is unique and that it has been critical to accelerated retinal care.

"He's an engineer and a surgeon," Papac said. "That's rare. But he's immersed in the surgical environment on an almost daily basis, where he is also thinking like an engineer. Somebody with that type of experience basis is unique. He seems to always be thinking way ahead of a problem, and then he sends us a memo, we file a patent, and create a product out of it. He's just always been very effective at getting right to the point when it comes to what it takes to do something, and he can come up to speed on state of the art in a number of fields of engineering very quickly. I don't know of anyone else with both his understanding and passion."

As the Ocutome 8000 began to move into the medical marketplace for Coopervision, Charles was still thinking about improving the vitreous cutter. Probably no other tool on the surgical platform was more critical. The probe that entered the eye through the tiny cannula incision needed to cut quickly and avoid the winding of the fibrous vitreous, which could pull on the retina and cause further detachment. Increasing the cutting speed promised to improve efforts to safely and effectively reattach retinas. Charles was also concerned about the weight and the shape of vitreous cutters. They were mostly awkward to hold, which affected a surgeon's hand movement inside of the eye, and appeared to lack the precision required for vitreoretinal operations.

Because their collaboration for Coopervision on the Ocutome 8000 had been successful, Charles and Wang decided to form a company called MidLabs and to develop a new type of cutter that might serve as the foundation of yet another advanced surgical platform. Using as a model the electric-driven solenoid axial cutter developed by eye surgery innovator Gholam Peyman, which used a guillotine motion and reduced the problem of winding vitreous, they considered a potentially improved design. Peyman's vitreous tool had been invented at about the time the Ocutome 800 was launched, but it was not incorporated into that platform because Conor O'Malley and Ralph Heinz already had a cutter they had engineered.

The goal of MidLabs was to design and manufacture a self-sharpening, affordable, and even disposable vitreous cutter. Charles incorporated the new company in Tennessee and raised the capital to launch production, but operations were located in California with Wang. Charles concentrated on designing an hourglass-shaped cutter that was lighter and more comfortable in the hand. It could be disposed of after surgery and was more functional than the slower, reusable vitreous cutters circulating in operating rooms.

The tool, called the MicroVit, was pneumatic driven and was central to a surgical platform that employed a linear foot pedal that managed a vacuum, an air pump, an integrated light source, power instruments like scissors and forceps, a fragmenter, and an electrocautery. Even before MidLabs managed to bring on a sales staff, Charles had sold 105 of the new units. The various elements of the platform became basic to the retinal surgery machines that were designed and manufactured in the coming decades.

"I was at the beginning of a process where I learned that I didn't like business as much as engineering and helping people to see," Charles said. "I'd had a bad experience with my retina business partner in Memphis, and we'd parted ways. I felt like I was on an endless search to find the right business approach. I kind of thought that if I took money from industry that it was tainted. But I needed to build the things that I knew our profession needed. I just wasn't there yet with the optimal plan of how to do it commercially."

The market, however, *was* ready. As three-port vitrectomy became the standard of care for retinal surgery, demand increased for lighter, more functional, and precise tools to operate inside the eye. In a few short years, the MicroVit was so popular that MidLabs was acquired by medical manufacturing giant Alcon Laboratories. The platform was rebranded as the MVS System and began to take over a global market share. The sale, however, was managed in a manner that left Charles feeling he had not been properly treated financially. Charles had been pushing the deal and negotiating with Alcon, and he had a small venture firm that was about to earn a decent finder's fee. Unfortunately, no money was paid to him for constructing and closing the transaction, and Charles decided to no longer work with Wang, who had joined Alcon.

Instead, he started a new business called InnoVision.

On the flight home from Israel, Charles became convinced that the platform he had envisioned at the conference was the next evolutionary step for vitreoretinal surgeries, and he was already making plans to begin designing prototypes and manufacturing.

Rather than simply developing handheld tools driven by various power sources and fluidics, Charles wanted to bring diverse functionalities together into the single OCM system. His new platform, simple to use, would employ all his latest techniques and technology.

With the OCM, Charles said, "What I was trying to do was provide an integrated-systems solution to the vitreoretinal surgeon. What I understood was that the surgeon had to deal with various components, multiple foot pedals, and putting things together to get things done with tubing and wires. These are the things they had to use to accomplish their surgical goals. It seemed unnecessarily complicated and challenging."

Success with any vitreoretinal surgery platform always seemed to begin with advancing the tiny cutter that was inserted into the eye to chop up and aspirate the fibrous vitreous. The MVS cutters were driven by a diaphragm with a spring return; the diaphragm bowed inward, pushed a guillotine cutter, and then sheared the vitreous tissue. Speed was limited with these types of designs.

Charles wanted different mechanics on the OCM cutter.

"I wanted to design something that would work well with all of the new fluidics driving the surgical platform," he explained. "Doctors needed something that was lightweight and cheap enough to be disposable. It would be more efficient if it were driven by a dual actuated, reciprocating, transverse piston (InnoVit) instead of a bellows (Ocutome) or spring return diaphram (MidLabs). I liked the idea of a disposable dual actuation cutter with an hourglass-shaped handle. That's what I went to work on."

The doctor who did not want to be a businessman, Charles was again becoming just that. InnoVision, his little start-up, appeared poised to take on Alcon. Charles needed capital, however, and he began to evangelize his new company, its products, and their potential. He was looking for investors at an Aspen Retinal Detachment Society gathering during the mid-1980s when he encountered his former business partner. Carl Wang introduced him to Barry Caldwell, a senior executive at Alcon, and the two arranged a marketing agreement for InnoVision and the OCM.

The business challenge for Charles was not just the manufacturing process, the marketing, and growing of a market share as an independent engineering company. Charles had always hated raising money and dealing with investors and boards. The doctor's motivation had always been in ideas and treatment of patients. But as an engineer, the conception, design, and engineering of a surgical system energized him in the same manner as fixing a damaged retina and giving someone their eyesight back. Charles realized his inventions faced uncertain futures without the same detailed effort to business that he employed in surgery.

Jorge Calzada, a talented vitreoretinal surgeon who became Charles' partner in their successful practice in Memphis, said he often has to find a way to work around the doctor's dislike of managing money and business.

"I think dealing with money just makes Steve feel dirty," Calzada said. "He knows how important it is, but he has no interest in seeing any financial reporting. I swear you can almost see his skin crawl when he is given a financial report. It's kind of amusing. You place dollar signs in front of him, and his eyes glaze over. He loves to talk about business concepts, and he understands them well, but when you get into the data and details and why certain decisions are being made, he just doesn't want to deal with that. The summary of the information is enough for Steve most of the time. Of course, with his level of intelligence, that is usually enough."

Regardless of his dislike of business, Charles had always managed to overcome obstacles, and nothing was likely to stop him from succeeding with the OCM. The doctor had synthesized a concept that had the promise to be transformative to retinal surgery. He was excited and convinced he would get the OCM into the marketplace, and it would be a great success.

But there were complications not even a great visionary could see.

NINE

Darkness Risible

"So, you're back again?" the nurse asked.

"I'm afraid I am."

"You know we don't give frequent flyer miles here, don't you?"

"If you did, I'd be buying my own hospital right now."

A pleasant and attractive middle-aged woman, she laughed and said she would return shortly when they were ready to take me back for my surgery. The anesthesiologist entered my curtained room and asked what arm I wanted to use for my IV. When he had slipped the needle into my vein, I reminded him I had asked for a pre-op "cocktail" for relaxation. I had so little exposure to hospitals that I found myself as nervous as the days when I toed the starting line in a high school mile race.

"Got it right here," he said and held up a small syringe, which he plugged into my IV line. "You should feel pretty great, pretty fast."

Boy, was he right.

The almost instant euphoria made me understand drug addiction. A certain type of person might spend the rest of their lives chasing such a physical and psychological joy. Suddenly, it seemed the troubled world was a lovely place, everyone was wonderful, and the universe was beautiful. And even though I had but one eye after more than a year of surgeries and might not ever see out of it again, that concern was secondary to how I suddenly felt after the injection of a narcotic.

Before this new procedure, I had wanted to understand why I was not seeing after the previous operations to reattach my retina. A follow-up visit with Dr. D revealed my retina had detached a second time. Now, the situation had worsened to include my macula, the center of the eye's field of perception and the area of greatest visual acuity. How this had happened, Dr. D did not know. I had followed postoperative instructions with obsessive diligence.

"There was a bullous retinal detachment, which involved the macula," wrote Dr. D in his surgical documentation report for the hospital. "The superior temporal area was still attached with retinopexy around the previously healed tear."

Ordinarily, that second sentence would be good news. The laser Dr. D had used to perform retinopexy—reattaching the retina at the location of the previous tear—was still holding. Unfortunately, I now had this bullous detachment that involved the most important part of my eye, and he had no readily available explanation for the cause.

"The truth is, Mr. Moore," he said, "we don't really know what might cause a detachment. Holes appear, inexplicably, in the retina, fluid leaks, and there is detachment. But many retinas have holes and nothing happens. The retina sometimes just separates from the rest of your eye without trauma or any immediately understandable explanation. It could be genetics. We just don't know for certain, and each case is relatively different."

I certainly did not like how "different" my case was becoming.

The previous two procedures, one in Dr. D's office and the other in a hospital operating room, had both failed to keep my retina attached. The plan for this third attempt was to inject silicone oil into my eye and leave it there for some time, while the retina was held in place by the surface tension of the oil. Because no hole or tear had caused the current detachment around the macula, Dr. D was forced to make an incision in the retina to remove subretinal fluid. Called a drainage retinotomy, the opening enabled him to use an extrusion cannula to withdraw fluid behind the detachment, which made the retina move back into its proper position. He applied endolaser, and I was back in recovery.

The use of silicone oil for a problem retina was both troubling and hopeful. As long as the substance remained in my eye, I was less likely to suffer another detachment. I had heard that many people saw through the oil almost as clearly as if it were vitreous, but for me the light was refracted and images distorted. The first time I looked at the digital display on my truck radio at night, I noticed the numbers and letters were slanted and crooked. There was no way to correct the distortion, which was similar to a very bad astigmatism. There was also now definitely a risk of redetachment caused by a possible epiretinal membranes (ERM) with increased traction on the retina. ERM membranes are a kind of scar tissue on the retina and can make it impossible for the retina to remain attached. The complications and odds of failure for my eye were increasing with each operation.

The oil was expected to remain in my eye at least three months. Actually, my research had taught me that the average time was just over a year before doctors were comfortable with removal. More than 10 percent of retinas treated by silicone oil detach again on extraction of the oil. The surface-tension management properties of the oil are often the only force keeping the retina attached, and for reasons of varying pathophysiology, it simply does not always reattach over time. Use of the oil also carried risks, including cataracts and glaucoma as well as redevelopment of recurrent ERM (i.e. PVR).

I was impatient to have the oil removed almost from the time I left the hospital. My willingness to wait might have been less filled with angst if my vision were not completely distorted with twisted images, wavy lights, and fluttering movement that was impossible to track. Unfortunately, I trusted my body and my health more than was logical. After a couple of operations, I ought to have gotten a clue that maybe my healing was not as easy as it had been with cuts and broken limbs. I assumed that in a few months my retina would certainly be reattached after having silicone oil hold it in position for that period of time.

"Your healthiness might be a part of the problem," Dr. D told me. "Your body would appear to have a strong healing response, which leads to complicated cell growth on the retina, obscuring vision, thickening the surface, and making detachment more likely each time you begin the healing process."

As hard as it was to understand, healing was actually a problem. Science has found no way to moderate the growth of cells as the body heals from injury. The system's natural reaction is to send blood and nutrition to rejuvenate what has been hurt. This means that many of the complications that arise after retinal detachments are the consequence of too much healing-related cellular growth. ERMs proliferate and have to be peeled to reattach the retina.

My immediate problem, however, was a recurrence of strabismus; my right eye was wandering. There might have been a number of reasons. Scleral buckles can cause strabismus but so can a lack of vision as the eye struggles to focus and see. Every potential cause was manifested in my case, and I began to wear a patch again to see if rest would cause the eye to move properly and track with the healthy one. I was very self-conscious about how distracting my cross-eyed appearance was to other people, which was another reason for putting on the eye patch again. The affliction also kept me from engaging my consulting clients in person, and the lack of contact began to affect my income.

In any case, it was spring in Texas, and, of course, I wanted to play baseball. The notion was unrealistic and a bit stupid. An increasingly monocular man ought to have enough sense to not put his good eye in jeopardy. I had no business exposing my healthy eye to incoming pitches. Admittedly, we did not have Major League fastballs sizzling over the plate in the Men's Senior Baseball League in Austin. But there were still athletes with college experience, a few with minor league backgrounds, and players in their 40s who often threw as high as 80 mph, a velocity sufficient to knock loose the other retina if I took one to the head.

But I loved baseball.

A friend had given me the advice to live my life as if nothing had yet happened to me, which I wanted to follow as wise counsel, but it was absurd. Watching the baseball come at me during a spring practice left me with no doubt that I had undergone a change. My vision was never great, but with corrective lenses I saw the baseball spin and was able to calculate location with decent accuracy as it approached the plate. Gauging speed and watching the ball rotate increased the odds of contact. However, a dysfunctional eye ruined depth of field. The ball seemed to come upon me much more quickly, and I felt as though I were swinging almost at the same time I heard the thud in the catcher's mitt.

And then came the jokes.

"Hey, we're the River Dogs," my coach yelled. "Not the Pirates. Lose the patch."

"You wouldn't like what you saw under it," I said.

"Okay, but it seems like you aren't making contact with the ball while you're wearing that."

"Ha, yeah, well, that's the heart of the problem. Not exactly a matter of choice to wear it right now. I hope my brain adjusts."

"Me too. But what about your fielding at first?"

"I guess I'll find out."

Lovers of the game often view fielding a baseball as an art. The most skilled practitioners can make the snagging of a speeding and skidding ball look routine. The fielder begins, when possible, by squaring his shoulders up against the oncoming ball. With knees bent slightly, he's poised to jump upward, move right or left with a quick step, lunge, or dive. His glove is always pointed down to make certain the ball does not slip beneath it on a short skip, and the bare hand is held above the open webbing to secure the ball once it arrives in the leather. Infielders' abilities vary based upon the countless hours they have had a coach or friend hit grounders in their direction or how many games they've played. No one comes to the talent with natural ease.

Depth perception is critical for fielding ground balls, and I suddenly lacked it. As a left-handed man, six feet two inches tall, I generally found myself playing first base. Baseball protocol assumes that when the batter is left-handed, the first baseman will back up a few steps because he needs a second more to adjust to the speed of the ball. He's still close enough to the base to have adequate time to field the ball and reach the base before the runner. The standard approach, however, did not work for me my first time on a diamond with only one good eye.

The coach began slapping some slow ground balls in my direction near the first base bag, and I immediately struggled. Instead of keeping my glove low and ready and moving it fluidly in the direction of the baseball, I found that it took longer to determine where it was going. I ended up stabbing at the ball late, sometimes after it had passed. In fact, as the coach began to hit the ball harder, and it moved directly toward me, I began to worry. If the ball were to take an awkward bounce toward my chest or my head, I realized, I might not be able to knock it down or take a protective position. The coach noticed my reticence and lack of capability and hit the ball a bit more easily in my direction. I caught a few, but it was clear things had changed. My confidence as a fielder was gone in a matter of minutes.

I knew what had caused the difference, but I was unable to accept my condition. To have played baseball with some degree of skill and confidence and then to have lost it for reasons beyond one's control is almost psychologically debilitating. One eye did not process depth of field as quickly and efficiently as two, and I wondered if it would ever be possible to see that way with a solitary eye. A fair amount of research about the brain showed that it grew new neural pathways when certain parts of the body failed—a process called plasticity—and I began to read about how the brain processes information through one eye. Settled science proved that the brain could be taught or trained to improve the imagery it processes. If this were my straw to grasp at hope, I intended to hang onto it tightly.

When I was a boy, baseball had been my reason for existing. I had found an old glove when I was six or seven years old and clung to the thin leather, restringing the fingers with old shoelaces when the ties wore out and broke. We played catch under the streetlight in front of our house on warm summer nights in Michigan until our arms were too tired for even soft toss. Then, we went to bed and dreamed about the diving catches we might make on the craggy, weedy field in back of the neighborhood where many southern families had formed a factory workers' community.

I watched baseball on those rare days it was on the television—always the Detroit Tigers—and was never far from a radio when a game was being played and the voices of George Kell and Ernie Harwell filled the air. In the summer, on days when our Little League team had games, we rose with the sun and played catch in the backyard, trying to get loose prior to our start time, which was often six to eight hours later. I am pretty sure I have never loved anything that much since those days of youth baseball.

I gave up the game in my penultimate year before high school graduation, and it was an agonizing decision. The realization that I was simply too thin and not strong enough to get a baseball scholarship was a terrible truth to confront. Although I consistently got the bat on the ball, it rarely traveled far. Perhaps, with some adult guidance, I might have arrived at a different decision and been encouraged to lift weights and be patient with my growth, but I wanted to go to college, and a scholarship was necessary for that. Finally, at one point, I looked at my ectomorph frame and realized that I was better suited to be a runner.

After switching to cross-country and track, I found success, won long-distance races, and began to interest colleges and universities. I entered university on a scholarship and kept up a rigorous and disciplined training regimen, running down country roads on Michigan's cold, snowy mornings. But I did not stop dreaming of warm afternoons in baseball stadiums, chasing line drives along the foul line, getting key hits, and dancing down the dugout steps as the hero of the day. Instead, I drifted into a career in broadcast journalism and on weekends played fast-pitch softball before I eventually ended up in slow-pitch beer leagues. Those softball contests, especially the co-ed teams, did not satisfy my need for competition. I didn't care for the larger ball, shorter base paths, and closer fences, and I simply stopped playing for many years.

When a new baseball league began expanding across the country, I rediscovered playing the game. At the age of 48, and after three decades of not even touching a baseball, I was again standing at first base, acting like not a minute had transpired since the last time I had played. I still knew the movements and situations and where to throw the ball. And the feeling of the ball in the glove after chasing down a hard-hit grounder was as satisfying as it had been when I was a teenager. When I finally made a perfect connection with a fastball, I knew it was headed for the fence, because I could not feel the ball hit the bat.

The time went fast, though, as it always does, and soon I was 60 years old, wearing a baseball mitt on a team that was considerably younger. My legs were still strong, though, I was fast, and I could make plays on the ball. I suppose love in all its manifestations can prompt bad judgment, but with ibuprofen, cold beer, and a few days' rest between games, I was hoping to keep playing. So there I was, taking ground balls while wearing an eye patch.

"Hey, why don't you go take some batting practice?" Coach Mike asked.

"Uh, yeah, okay, I just wanted to get comfortable around here."

"Yeah, but it doesn't look like you are," he said. "You are kind of poking at the ball with your glove hand. Do you see it okay?"

"Gets on me fast. I'm adjusting."

"Go take some swings."

Hitting with one eye felt considerably more natural than fielding.

My left eye, always dominant, faced the pitcher, and I felt like I could see the ball's spin and its release well enough to track its course and make contact. After a few pitches, I stroked maybe a half-dozen line drives into outfield gaps, not deep but in spots where they would have earned extra bases. The pitcher was not throwing with game-day speed, but he was not doing soft toss, either. I was happy, and I asked him to give me his "cheese." When he did, I still made solid contact, though not with much authority. I figured I simply needed to make some adjustments to my swing or position, which would come with more batting practice.

"What's the prognosis on your eye?" Coach Mike asked.

"Not sure. It's a detachment, pretty common. I'm healthy. Should be okay."

"You think you can play before it's back to 100 percent?"

"I'll take the extra hours of infield," I said. "I enjoy that."

"Your hitting doesn't seem to have suffered."

"No, I was pretty pleased. I actually felt like my astigmatism in the bad eye affected how well I saw pitches, so it might have helped with hitting."

"Well, maybe you shouldn't worry so much about getting it back then."

"Like hell," I said.

The coach walked away, and I spent another 90 minutes having my pal Kenny hit me infield ground balls. I don't think I ever got comfortable, though. The sun was Texas strong, and sweat stung my good eye to the point where I decided to quit. Ken and I had a cold beer but did not talk much; he knew what I feared, and there was no point in either of us articulating what it might be like to live without baseball. I could not avoid those thoughts, but that did not mean I needed to dwell on them. It would have been like talking about a death in the family.

Halfway through the three-month wait for silicone removal from my eye, I had another appointment with Dr. D. I struggled to maintain optimism as I drove to his office. After multiple bad visits, I had developed an almost physical nausea in response to the sight of his building. There was nothing good to report when he looked into my eye.

"I'm afraid you have a cataract," he said. "You need to see a cataract surgeon and get an artificial lens put in your eye."

"What's the point, if the retina isn't working?"

"I can't see through to determine if you are healing or what steps we need to take next. I can get an idea with the ultrasound, but I really need to see, and right now looking into your eye is like looking through a heavily frosted window."

"Great. How did I all of a sudden get a cataract?"

"Surgeries to the eye are traumatic, Mr. Moore. That trauma often causes the lens to cloud. I think your capsule is also clouded and scarring."

"What's my capsule again?"

"Sort of a clear bag of tissue that separates the front of your eye from the back. Your cataract surgeon will probably need to take a laser and cut that capsule open during your lens replacement."

I left with a referral to "the best cataract guy in Austin." As I walked across the parking lot, I looked up at the high, clear spring sky of Central Texas, and all I could think about was how hard it would be to track fly balls against that infinite blue.

TEN

Last Light

In 1986, eight-year-old Mark Mullen was hiding from the light. An aggressive benign tumor was growing in his right eye and causing uveitis, an inflammation of the tissues of the eye that prompted a sensitivity to light. The tumor, which was releasing protein that created scar tissue and fibrosis on the retina, was simply another visual complication for the boy. His eyesight had been deteriorating from the day he was born. There was also the pain. Mullen was taking so many medications that he spent much of his early boyhood curled up in a ball and sleeping on the couch. His latest issue was that the protein secreted by the benign tumor had caused his retina to become completely detached, and he was without vision in the eye.

"I came out of the womb with eye problems," Mullen told me more than three decades later. "My umbilical cord was wrapped around my neck, so there was some kind of oxygen-supply problem, and then that led to a misdiagnosis. I may have not had enough oxygen at birth for my eyes to be healthy, or the doctors might have responded the wrong way and gave me too much of an oxygen supplement. There's no real way to know."

Mullen's diagnosis, ultimately, was identified as retinal angioma, which causes the proliferation of random, disorganized capillary growth and new blood vessels that leak protein to cause scarring, retinal detachment, and a dramatic degradation of vision. Mullen also suffered from strabismus—a wandering eye.

When Mullen was still a baby, his family got a referral to Steve Charles to seek treatment. Though they lived near Memphis, they had never heard of the doctor, and no one yet knew the extent of the child's problems, but they had been told Charles might be able to help. The doctor often saw as many as 60 patients in one day, and Mark and his mother sat for hours in Charles' crowded office, waiting for the boy's turn to be examined.

"He really does want to help as many people as he can," Mullen said. "But we were unprepared for the wait. My mother ran out of diapers, and I was tired and cranky and wouldn't sleep. A nurse called us back for preliminary examination, and the first thing she did was shine a light in my eyes. I was none too happy and started crying. My mother was not impressed with Dr. Charles either."

Mullen's parents later took their son to a different optometrist and ophthalmologist for second opinions. The other doctors told Mullen's parents there was a serious problem developing in his right eye, though they offered no detailed prognosis or cure.

The Mullens had no intention of returning to the Charles Retina Institute until a dinner guest persuaded them. The woman was a technician at Charles' office, and she told Mullen's mother that her son was much too young to be wearing such strong corrective lenses.

Charles agreed to see the boy on a Saturday morning, when no other patients were in his office and at no cost to Mullen's family.

But early in his examination the doctor knew that the eye was going to have long-term problems.

"The root cause of the disorder," Charles said, "is incredible proliferation of these aggressive vessels, and the vessel walls are highly permeable. Protein exudates just pour through them and get under the retina and create membranes. We don't have the ability to control the basic process of this disease. Mark's situation is very unusual, and I've only managed a handful of them in my life."

Young Mullen's condition kept getting progressively worse. It seemed like darkness was closing in on him. Laser could be used to stop some of the capillaries from spreading and bleeding, but the protein and scarring overwhelmed any treatment plan devised by Charles. Mark remembered being in grade school and having an appointment at Charles Retina Institute when the doctor's assistant, Sabrina Newsom, put a light in his right eye and saw a "starburst" of blood and adhesions. Mullen's memory of sight in that eye is mostly tinged with fear.

"I remember being scared," he said. "I hadn't really been able to see out of that eye much anyway. But, you know, the darker it became, the more afraid I was. Any memory I have out of that eye is very young and blurry. I have memories of sitting around in the kitchen and closing my good eye and looking at my Flintstones vitamins on the counter, and it was really just a blurry white object."

Though Mullen developed a close, trusting relationship with the doctor, unfortunately, none of Charles' most advanced medical procedures or medicines were able to stop his vision's deterioration. All available treatments were failing. And Mullen's pain was increasing. Finally, at the age of eight, the boy faced a terrible choice.

"I was too young to know, I guess, how dire my situation was," Mullen said. "I just know I was in this constant pain, and I couldn't see out of the eye anyway. I just wanted the pain out of my head, and there was only one way that was going to happen. There really wasn't any choice to make."

The boy's eye needed to be surgically removed.

And many years later, his crisis and his courage would profoundly affect me.

THE PURPOSE OF InnoVision, like all of Charles' ideas, was to solve a problem. Making money was essential for the survival of a business, but for the doctor, it was secondary. The idea for the Ocular Connection Machine (OCM) seemed to claw at his mind. There were simply too many individual elements in the operating room for retinal surgeons to master and control using multiple devices. Charles thought the array of pedals on the floor looked almost like what confronted an organ player.

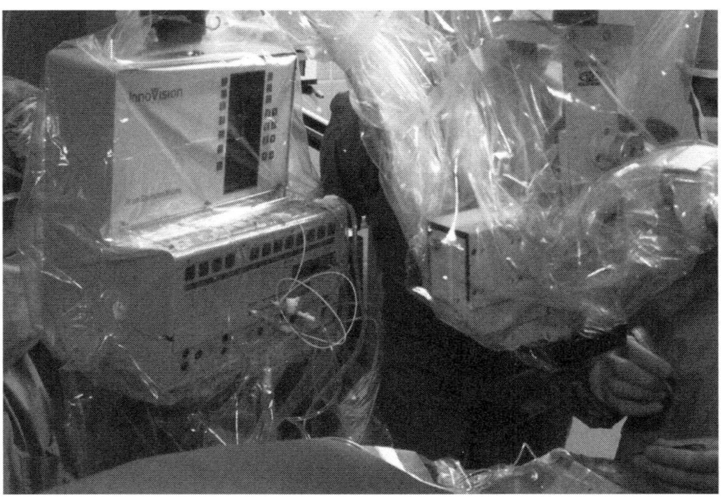

Ocular Connection Machine in operating room

"If you look at everything in the operating room," he said, "there seemed to be 10 different things made by 10 different companies. There was the MVS and then the light source and then the cautery and the air pump to infuse air into the eye. I just thought you needed to have all these things together and have one smart key graphical user interface and a switchable foot pedal. I was the first to integrate these functions into a single machine."

He was not the only one trying to resolve the complications inherent in the abundance of devices and tools in the operating room. The Storz Instrument Company was working to integrate the various functions of retinal surgery into a solitary platform. The "Daisy" system was brought to the market as a "thoroughly integrated unit" that used a modified version of Charles' MicroVit cutter and included irrigation, aspiration, anterior and posterior vitrectomy, bipolar coagulation, automated scissors, illumination, air pump, phacoemulsification, and fragmentation.

Charles, meanwhile, had been hard at work on his OCM, which was to be sold to vitreoretinal surgeons by his InnoVision company. There was clearly going to be competition in the marketplace, but Storz had already recognized the quality of Charles' MicroVit vitreous cutter and built the Daisy platform around the latest version even as the doctor was inventing another and more advanced vitreous cutter. In fact, the range of capabilities were broad enough that the platform could have been considered a certain low-risk success for investors. Charles and one other retinal surgeon evaluated the OCM in the operating room because virtually every functionality they needed existed on the platform, and they wanted to test performance before going to market.

"The OCM had a xenon light source, servo-controlled intraocular pressure (IOP), global functions, a smart key graphical user interface, tool ID, a tubing management system incorporated into a sterile patient interface, the dual-actuation InnoVit (no spring), 1,500 cuts per minute, push prime, and proportional diathermy, all of which are implemented on more refined and later platforms like the Alcon Constellation. The Constellation uses RFID instead of the more primitive tool ID system on the OCM, but the OCM began the revolution of system integration, a steadily increasing number of functions in one console under unified control using a graphical user interface and smart keys."

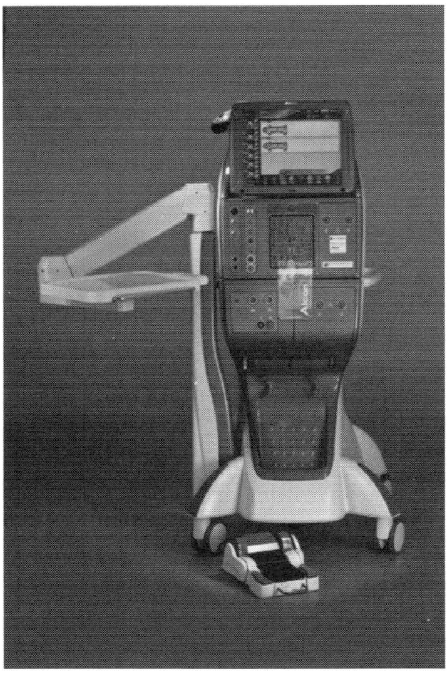

The Constellation Surgical System

Because of Charles' reputation and the infusion of some of his own capital, InnoVision got attention for its prospective surgical inventions and, with an engineering team of about 100 people, enjoyed quick growth. The doctor was trying to build a company, raise investment capital to sustain research and development of the OCM, and stay on top of his field as a surgeon. These endeavors were not necessarily compatible, even for a person with Charles' intellectual heft and abundant energy, especially since he preferred treating patients to launching a business.

"The problem with start-ups," Charles said, "is not just the need to go around begging for money from private equity investors. It has also always been challenging to get the right managers: Somebody who exaggerates his skill set or works 30 hours per week is not going to make it happen. I don't like begging for money, and I don't like sorting through managers who don't manage well. The problem with the medical-device industry is well known now. Anybody can get an MBA and an engineering degree and claim to have accomplished a paradigm shift, but they really only copy existing technology and become another 'me too' company."

Regardless of his personal ambivalence about business, Charles was making the adjustments necessary to grow his manufacturing company, improve retinal surgery, and earn revenue. The Storz Instrument Company, which was also working on its retinal surgery platforms, had begun to get customers using that altered version of the MicroVit cutter. Charles and his MidLabs executives were having conversations with Storz about acquiring the company, but the deal never transpired. When Alcon bought MidLabs, though, Charles was freed to begin work on realizing his dream of creating the Ocular Connection Machine through InnoVision.

Investors were interested in InnoVision and the OCM because of Charles' leadership and his previous successes with invention and engineering. He had already created the first disposable cutter in the MicroVit, which had the more comfortable hour-glass shape that fit well in the hands of surgeons and kept them from tiring so fast from a tight grip. The MicroVit had helped to drive Alcon's purchase of MidLabs. The OCM and an even more advanced InnoVit cutter had obvious potential to prospective investors in medical devices. Charles had agreed to terms with a Midwestern venture capital firm called Norwest Ventures early in the development of the OCM and InnoVision. That relationship foundered, however, when Norwest Ventures brought in a new partner.

"I thought we had a good deal that would benefit both parties," Charles said. "But they brought in a new partner to be on our board, and there seemed to be an immediate culture clash. We were due for another round [of financing] for the OCM, and [the partner] told me that if I didn't personally match their investment, he would not approve putting their money in. He just said, 'I am your new venture partner, and I don't like medical devices.'"

Charles took the call from the new partner during a board meeting at InnoVision headquarters in California just before the Christmas holidays. When the call ended, he said, "I'm out of here." The doctor got into his car and drove to Alcon's R&D offices, and began telling them more about his OCM, although a marketing agreement was already in place. Charles met with Bill Freeman, the general manager of the company's Irvine Technology Center. Freeman had joined Alcon after early successes in developing and marketing cataract surgical systems and devices, and he was known as an innovative thinker on prospective technology.

"I told Bill Freeman the OCM was ready," Charles recalled. "And he picked up the phone and called Barry Caldwell, who I had met at the retina conference in Aspen. He told Caldwell, 'We need this machine. Let's buy it.' They fairly quickly made a deal to acquire the OCM from InnoVision for the engineering and development work we had put into it. The VC firm was bought out. But I made zero; I received no money in the deal that was put together and no royalty because it was acquired."

Still, there were advantages. First, Charles had connected with the Alcon visionaries who believed in his machine and in him. Second, someone else would deal with the long, tedious slog involved in bringing medical innovation to market. Federal government approvals are often required for systems testing, and a final sign-off by the Food and Drug Administration is needed before a single unit of anything can be sold, in most cases. Bringing surgical platforms or devices to the consumer is not possible without long-term commitments to a vision plus the capital essential for creation of the final product. Although Charles had already invested several years and millions of dollars in his project, the remaining technical and financial challenges would still be intimidating to *any* entrepreneur. That is why he pursued the deal with Alcon.

Alcon's decision to buy the OCM from InnoVision was a critical move that was to have a significant impact on the company's fortunes. There were two great risks at the time of acquisition, and they were hardly minor. The costs of the OCM made its market reach prohibitive. Charles' platform used the new dual-actuation disposable InnoVit cutter, and the early iterations were pricey, limiting the number of buyers for the OCM. The move was further complicated by the fact that Storz had brought out its Daisy platform. Though its capabilities and functionalities were not, initially, drawing widespread adoption, the company would later become a part of eye-care giant Bausch & Lomb, which could provide great marketing power.

Alcon, also, was in a relatively precarious financial position at the time it acquired InnoVision. The company had moved into the production of surgical devices, and its emerging product line was, as executives admitted, "not that well done, and second rate." The Alcon front office was committed, however, to "getting it right," even though vitreoretinal surgery revenues in the late 1980s were only around $10 million annually, and investments in major projects like the OCM were fraught with peril. The central risk was the time needed for development and a return on investment, something that was also likely to frustrate Charles, who was accustomed to deciding and then acting.

In the end, the OCM's features and technology were incorporated into new products for Alcon.

Paul Hallen, the global director of retina for Alcon, nevertheless knew the company was making an important move by bringing Charles into its fold; there was no other comparable surgeon-engineer with both clinical and technical insights.

"Even though the OCM never became a product for us," he said, "it was the forerunner of some very big things. Working with Steve, we developed Accurus and then Constellation, the surgical platforms that dominated the market in retina. He consulted for us and helped us generate ideas that led to a portfolio of projects with integrated systems needed for eye surgery. That $10 million revenue grew by hundreds of millions working with Steve Charles, and Alcon is still collaborating with him. He's just a great retina specialist who approaches his job in an engineering fashion, and every surgical maneuver he does, he is thinking about ideas for managing the forces working on the retina."

Technology was beginning to transform more than medicine in the '80s, and the emergence of integrated circuits and basic computer functionalities for consumer products were trends that fired Charles' inventiveness. Dr. Robert Laborde, who was a fellow at the Charles Retina Institute during that time, marveled at the accomplishments and influence of his mentor across three decades.

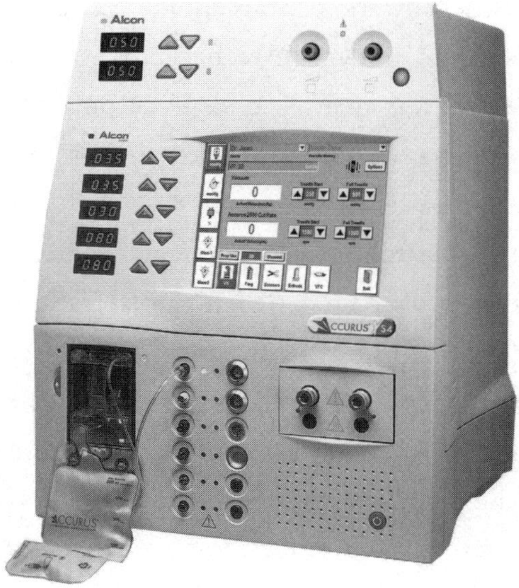

The Accurus Surgical System

"When [Robert] Machemer first put instruments into the eye," he said, "you have to understand it was Steve who got that fine-tuned with a foot pedal so that we could control how much vacuum was applied to the vitreous and scar tissue. In the early days, a cannula pumped fluid in with continuous-infusion pressure control, and it's hard to overestimate how huge that is. Every retinal surgeon in the world takes for granted that the eye stays pumped up, and those very precise moves are all possible because of the engineering he brought to it. I think it is reasonable to say Steve Charles has done for retina what Steve Jobs did for Apple and computing. But in this case, Steve is actually [Steve] Wozniak."

Charles, despite his disdain for raising money and placating investors, was an inveterate entrepreneur. He might have excelled simply as a technology innovator or software engineer or IT hardware designer and manufacturer. His understanding of what needed to be accomplished by the various tools of a surgical system was, indeed, analogous to leaders in technology giants like Apple and Microsoft. He, too, was creating tools to accomplish the tasks most valued by consumers, which, in his case, were retinal surgeons and hospitals with eye patients.

However, the research and development cycle of a retinal surgery platform is considerably longer than the latest iteration of a consumer device like an iPhone or the most recent MacBook, though none of these products is brought to the market without significant research and testing. One key difference is that Apple has remained in a market-share fight with Microsoft and PC users, while the Charles' vitreoretinal surgery systems, which continue to evolve, have gone on to dominate global markets.

That's mostly because Charles was as relentless in his determination to be a top engineer as he was the best possible retinal surgeon.

"I built a conceptual design of the Constellation with 1,200 parts in the proposed parts list before Alcon did one hour of work on it," he said. "I didn't sketch stuff on a napkin. I built a big computer-aided design (CAD) model with what the electronics should be, and the Constellation is built very much along those lines. Numerous technologies and patents on the Constellation come from me; same with the Accurus, and before that, the MVS and the Ocutome 8000."

Charles had many other ideas for products outside of retinal surgery, and he was already envisioning their design and manufacture. He saw himself having an impact on orthopedics and brain and spine surgery with new inventions, which he refined on a daily basis. The doctor was confident these inventions would make it to the market and help many people.

If only he could survive the business of being a businessman.

ELEVEN

The Man by the Side of the Road

Driving through the Mississippi countryside, Steve Charles was thinking about the talk he was going to give to students at the high school in Smithville. He had always been passionate about the idea that young people all had different capabilities and that many of them might have fulfilled lives without a college education. Charles was also hoping to inspire local educators and officials to do the work necessary to attract manufacturing facilities to their community and provide opportunities for their children to take advantage of technical training. Less than 1,000 people lived in Smithville, and the doctor was hoping that he might provide even a touch of inspiration that could prompt students and their parents to think differently about their community and their futures.

Charles had been invited to speak by a former patient, a man who had been shot in the face during a hunting accident. He had lost one eye, but Steve had been able to save the other. Though initially two or three people from his office were considering making the drive with the doctor, he ended up traveling alone. That was fine; Charles was fond of having quiet time to contemplate what he might do better as a father, surgeon, and engineer.

There was much for him to be professionally pleased about. The surgical platform that he had first envisioned as the Ocular Connection Machine (OCM) had made it to the international market under the brand name Accurus two years earlier, in 1997, after half a dozen years of development. It was now gobbling up market share for Alcon. Charles had become a consultant to the company after it had purchased his earlier technology, and he had worked with their engineers to realize the design and manufacture of the vitreoretinal surgery system that was making operations simpler and more efficient for doctors and increasing positive outcomes for patients. Charles was already sketching next-generation technological improvements.

The road was flat and empty and the weather mostly clear as Charles neared Smithville. Suddenly, an Oldsmobile Cutlass Sierra slammed into the doctor's Audi. The driver had run a stop sign traveling fast and got T-boned by Charles' car, blowing out the windows and blasting open all the doors and the trunk with the impact. Charles barely remembers the impact or the glass exploding and wheels screeching as they were pushed across the blacktop. When the two vehicles came to rest, they were in a pasture in a state of crumpled ruin. There had been four men in the Cutlass, and because they had not been wearing seat belts, two had been thrown almost 100 feet away; another was entangled in barbed wire, and the fourth lay in a drainage ditch at the side of the road.

As Charles regained his senses, he realized his right leg was broken, and pain of a few deep breaths indicated he also had some broken ribs. His first instinct, unsurprisingly, was to act as a doctor and assist the men who had almost cost him his life; the two who had been thrown so far were initially out of Charles' line of sight and ultimately died. Although he could barely walk, Charles made his way to the two men he could see. They were unconscious. He cleared their airways to make certain they could breathe until the arrival of emergency assistance. Then, he freed the man trapped in barbed wire and stabilized his neck, which appeared as if it had suffered severe injury.

The first two passers-by at the scene of the accident—the sheriff and Smithville's mayor—were both on their way to hear Charles speak. They immediately sent out calls to emergency services. The severity of the doctor's injuries prompted the EMT to ask for a helicopter to get him to Memphis, but storm clouds had built to the west, and weather threatened any flight. Instead, Charles was raced in a personal vehicle up the state highway to Baptist Memorial Hospital, the large private facility where he performed many of his vitreoretinal surgeries.

"I was admitted on a Monday," Charles said. "And I had scheduled 14 or 15 retinal surgeries for the very same hospital the next day. I always kept a Tuesday-and-Thursday operating schedule. They operated on my knee that Wednesday, a few days after the crash." He left the hospital on Saturday and the following Monday saw 65 patients at his office, while he was in a wheelchair.

When he went back to his surgical theater a week after being operated on for his injuries, Charles managed to operate on 16 vitreoretinal patients in one very long day. The pedals on the Accurus, which control various instruments in the eye and the operating microscope functions, were controlled with a single foot. Over the next weeks, as he healed, Charles thought about what had been said to him by visitors to his hospital suite during his recovery.

"I am friends with the tech guys at the hospital, and three of them stopped by to wish me well. Most everyone around the hospital had heard about the wreck. A couple of the tech guys asked me, 'You know why you ain't dead, Doc? You know why? Cause you ain't done with your work.'"

Although he had never been given to believe in notions like destiny and divine preordination, Charles might have wondered how he had survived several brushes with disaster. A motorcycle crash when he was a teenager in South Florida had broken his neck a week before his high school graduation. The Charles family lived in a grove of fruit trees, and Charles often rode his BSA Gold Star 500 down the dirt roads. When an old Ford Anglia pulled in front of him unexpectedly, he laid down the motorcycle and was thrown through the air. The landing resulted in a fracture of his C-6 vertebra and meant Charles had to lie in bed, in traction, for a week.

The next two times Charles broke his back, he was no longer a fearless teenager, and his great surgical skill was suddenly in jeopardy. In one accident, Charles was barefoot waterskiing with his family at 45 miles per hour. When he went to switch the towline from one hand to another, he lost his grip and fell so hard that one of his gloves flew 50 feet into the air. By the time the boat stopped moving, the doctor's arm was beginning to lose feeling and he was unable to move it.

Charles also was injured during a horseback-riding mishap. He had purchased a champion jumping horse and enjoyed the sport until the animal inexplicably stopped when approaching a four-foot fence. The doctor was thrown from the animal and landed on his C-7 vertebra, which aggravated his boyhood injury. Initially he simply felt "funny," but he was still able to operate on patients. Eventually, though, numbness set in, and he found he was unable to even lift his briefcase, which prompted a CT scan and an MRI.

"The scans found a fracture and what amounted to a notch in

my spinal cord," Charles said. "They did a cervical fusion and took a piece of bone from my hip to use in my neck. But, a week later, I could see patients, and I did my usual Tuesday-and-Thursday operating schedules without any problems."

The doctor physically recovered from all his injuries, though the collision in Mississippi had other lingering complications. The men who had intentionally run the stop sign decided to sue the doctor who had stabilized them and saved their lives. They wanted $10 million for his negligence in "failing to maintain a lookout." (The concept is generally applied to vessels operated in navigable waters but has been used as a novel legal assertion in motor-vehicle claims where there was an actual failure to adhere to traffic laws.) The plaintiffs lost the case but not without the waste of a lot of Charles' time and large legal bills to resolve a crisis in which he had been the victim. Investigators discovered the men were running stop signs intentionally as a form of Russian roulette, an absurd and dangerous game that cost two of them their lives.

Meanwhile, Charles' professional endeavors were all increasingly successful. The Charles Retina Institute in Memphis, which would later relocate to a new building in suburban Germantown, had become a center of learning and excellence that attracted the most critical patients and the brightest retinal surgeons seeking to become fellows and study under Charles. The business of improving vitreoretinal surgery remained an engineering challenge that never left his mind. He was convinced constant improvement was not only possible from an engineering perspective but also inevitable.

The vitreous cutter tended to be the focus of Charles' attention. In 1993, he had filed a patent with Alcon for a tool he had named the "InnoVit," reminiscent of his previous company's name, InnoVision. The device was an advancement of vitreous cutting because it altered the approach to removing the viscous substance from the eye more quickly, while also reducing the risk of traction on the retina and of creating worse detachments or more tears.

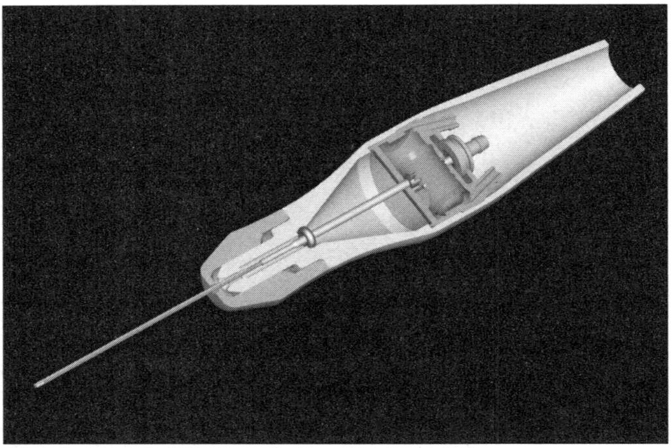

InnoVit Design Schematic, early Charles advancement to vitreous cutter

Charles called his new concept a dual-pneumatic drive. The state of the art for vitreous probes at the time involved using a large tank of compressed gas that was connected to a console with a single fast valve. Those pulses of gas pressure moved the cutter blade forward, and after it made the cut, a spring returned the blade to a "firing" position. The Charles design used pneumatic pressure from two valves and two lines to move the blade from side to side without a spring return.

As a result, the InnoVit delivered a dramatic increase in cutting speed. Previous vitreous tools were making 600–800 cuts per minute; that immediately doubled with the InnoVit. Those speeds would accelerate even more over the ensuing years, leading to a cutting speed of about 10,000 per minute on Alcon's Constellation Vision System. The greater the number of cuts, the less chance of pulling on the retina and better percentages of positive surgical results. Dual-pneumatic drive also gave surgeons more nuanced control over how long the port in the cutter remained open for cutting and aspiration of vitreous, which reduced inadvertent retinal tears.

Technological innovations like this in medicine tend to occur slowly for several reasons. The most obvious are the legal constraints that require government approvals for the use of new devices. An equally inhibiting factor is that engineers generally do not think like physicians, and doctors are generally not engineers. While both types of intellect are given to problem solving, they rarely occur within the mind of one individual, which is why Charles has an unequalled list of accomplishments and a reputation to match.

"What's most compelling about Steve is that he strikes a perfect balance between scientist and clinician," said Dr. Carl Regillo of the Wills Eye Hospital in Philadelphia. "Some of us are good scientists and innovators but aren't clinicians, and yet he manages to excel at both. There is no surgeon alive or who has ever lived, in my view, who has ever done as much as Steve has. The fact that the average surgeon can now manipulate retinal tissue that is just cells thick, and do it safely, says a great deal about what he has brought to the table."

What Charles has brought to the table is estimated to be worth well over $5 billion in sales, most of which went to Alcon, minus the royalties to the engineer-designer. The doctor has more than 100 patents issued or pending and continues to create technology, though he insists his work is about something more important than innovation.

"No, it's not about innovation," Charles said. "And it's not entrepreneurship. It's not about business. Again, it's about problem solving. And so it's constantly an overlap of what I call the three Ts: technique, technology, and teaching. If you don't do a ton of surgery, you're not valid in the design space. If you don't keep current in engineering, and push the envelope, and teach yourself things like mechatronics, modern control theory, field-programmable gate arrays (FPGAs), and photonics, like I've done, then you just aren't valid in the engineering domain."

The doctor might have added that patience was also essential. Although his patent on the InnoVit cutter was filed in 1993, the tool was not included in the launch of the Accurus platform because of strenuous and lengthy reliability testing. The InnoVit was added to the Accurus in 2001, four years after the surgical system had been made available for purchase. Even as the platform was already building a global reputation for reliability and improved surgical outcomes, Charles was working with Alcon on next-generation improvements, which became the Constellation Vision System.

The three most critical functions of a vitreoretinal surgery platform are what engineers call, bluntly, "cut, suck, and illuminate." Prior to the Accurus, there had never been a single machine that had all key functions integrated into one box, and the emergence of color-touch screen technology at the time of deployment gave surgeons a simple console to manage their delicate retinal operations. The Constellation added a solid state laser and xenon light source. Surgeons could now cut and aspirate vitreous tissue much faster with the new dual-actuation probe, control vacuum rates, brightly illuminate the interior of the eye while it was a surgical field, and perform any needed laser repairs to the retina.

Richard Lindstrom, M.D., a world-class corneal and cataract surgeon from Minnesota and a close associate of Charles, believes it is impossible to overstate the importance of the inventor's ideas.

"He sits in his office and sees a problem," Lindstrom said. "And then he goes home with his engineering mind, with all his training and years of experience, and he evolves a solution to the problem he sees in his practice. This is what he's been doing since he became a doctor. If there isn't a solution, and he comes up with one, Steve puts his money where his mouth is and often brings technology to the market before he is able to convince a larger company to launch it globally. But he doesn't just stop there. Steve keeps working to make his tools and devices better while he also goes out and teaches others how to use it. He impacts the profession and a total number of lives I don't think we can ever know or measure."

The surgical platforms that Charles helped design, build, and launch reduced the dangers of a physician's hands causing damage during microsurgery. There were also improvements that allowed a full range of visibility inside of the eye, enhancing the surgeon's work and the odds of a positive outcome for a patient. Nonetheless, human beings have limitations even with increased visibility and precision tools, and their ability to accurately diagnose what has happened in the intraocular space will always be constrained by experience and education. The next frontier for ophthalmology, and almost especially retinal surgery, is robotics and the type of technology that can analyze what is anatomically wrong with an eye and then perform most, if not all the surgical corrections.

Corneal transplant, cataract removal, and replacement of the cataractous lens have already become increasingly automated and robotic, along with the use of computer-guided lasers to reshape the front of the eye to improve vision. The question is how much of a delicate microsurgery like retinal repair can be turned over to automation and robotics. Bruno Dacquay, who has worked with Charles for many years while heading the surgical research and development division of Alcon, has said the technology is feasible. It just needs to be designed and built.

"There's no question we need technology that will detect anatomical disorders in the eye," Dacquay said. "And it should tell the physician what to fix. Currently, a surgeon relies on his own eyes. You need as much information as possible to guide surgery, and we should look at where we are with retinal surgery compared to where we have come from. What was a 2-hour surgery is now done in under 30 minutes, and it is performed with a microsurgical instrument of 27-gauge. The impact of the surgeon in the eye is considerably less than it was before. Cruder, earlier instruments did repair the retina, but there was frequently collateral damage. I see no reason we can't keep evolving our technology for the interior of the eye."

Increasingly, robotics is becoming central to surgical platforms for everything from brain and cancer surgery to orthopedics. Charles, predictably, has been interested in the specialty for decades, and not necessarily only for retinal surgery. His accomplishments in robotics are less well known than his others but are not without great merit. The doctor might have naturally turned his attention to this emerging industry, but, in fact, he did so because he was acting on a promise he had made years ago to his dying father.

And the record will show the doctor kept his word.

TWELVE

Eyes to the Sky

The giant MD-10 aircraft rolled slowly across the ramp at the Federal Express World Hub in Memphis. Two water cannons blasted glistening arches into the air, forming rainbows over the plane as it passed underneath. A slight turn to the right in front of the old Memphis airport terminal revealed lettering on the side of the fuselage. The small crowd of officials who had been invited to the aircraft's christening could easily read the words "Orbis" and "Flying Eye Hospital" painted in sky blue.

The year was 2016, and Orbis, an international organization that flies eye doctors and other medical professionals to the developing world, was unveiling its third-generation airborne hospital. A couple of days later, a larger group was invited to see the big jet that had been donated by Federal Express. The spectators would bear witness to this impressive convergence of aviation and ophthalmological technology, a state-of-the-art hospital designed as cargo modules and loaded into an aircraft that would deliver life-changing vision care.

Jack McHale, a former aircraft buyer for FedEx, watched the plane's slow approach with a private sense of fulfillment. He had spent six years working with the shipping giant, corporations, and private donors to raise the more than $30 million in cash and in-kind contributions to outfit the onboard surgical and teaching systems. McHale, who has the trim look of a retired professional golfer with thick gray hair and a healthy dose of California sun darkening his complexion, struggled to control his emotions when he was asked to speak.

"I believe that everyone who has been a part of the creation of the new Flying Eye Hospital should be very proud of the achievement," he said. "And while the aircraft is a marvel of aviation and medical ingenuity and resourcefulness, its purpose is what is most important. It is a transportation and delivery device. A tool that makes it possible for the dedicated medical staff to deliver the gift of sight to millions and millions of needlessly vision-impaired individuals around the world. This gift will transform lives from despair and desperation to ones of hope and promise."

Combating the pervasive visual impairment in the developing world was the rationale behind the launch of Orbis. The idea originated with David Paton, M.D., an ophthalmologist from a family of accomplished physicians. His father, Richard Townley Paton, M.D., had founded the world's first eye bank in 1946 to grow the practice of corneal transplants. David Paton conceived of flying eye doctors to remote parts of the world, and he began searching for surplus World War II aircraft that he might retrofit to launch his global eye-care charity. He had no luck on his own, but eventually, he remembered his childhood friend Betsy Trippe, the daughter of Pan American Airways founder Juan Trippe, and he asked her to see if her dad might provide an airplane.

The elder Trippe had no spare airplane for their charitable cause, but he sent Paton and his daughter to United Airlines. He also had his personal pilot, Al Ueltschi, accompany the pair in order to provide some aviation expertise as they made their case for a donated plane to United's CEO Ed Carlson. The story from that point forward might be apocryphal, but it has become the accepted version of corporate history in the Orbis offices.

Carlson is said to have denied the request for a large aircraft, but as the trio was leaving United's headquarters, Betsy looked up and saw an excerpt of a poem by Alfred Lord Tennyson hanging on the wall above the front desk. There was a reference to silver birds delivering hope, and she quoted the lines in a thank-you note she sent to Carlson. Betsy told the United CEO that it was his airline's destiny to give Orbis its first airplane. He apparently believed her, because a short time later, she and Paton were notified that Carlson was donating a DC-8 to the nascent charitable cause.

Ueltschi, who was also the founder and CEO of a global pilot-training company called Flight Safety, is credited as a co-founder of Orbis. At first, the problem Ueltschi wanted to address sounded overwhelming. Even today there remain, worldwide, an estimated 285 million people suffering from vision problems; four out of every five of them live with preventable conditions. Doctors estimate that 90 percent of these people live in countries with emerging economies and do not have access to sight-saving treatment. The task before Orbis was enormous. In 2015 alone, the organization performed 41,281 adult eye surgeries and 24,277 for children, while also offering 1,414 training courses for doctors in 92 different countries that advanced the skills of 30,326 medical professionals.

Yet, from the beginning, Ueltschi believed in the flying hospital concept as much as David Paton and Betsy Trippe did. Ueltschi raised money and solicited the support of physicians, and by 1982, a USAID grant and business donations enabled the organization to begin flying the DC-8, taking doctors and light equipment to places where people needed eye care. Because of the aircraft's size and lack of freight capacity, the Flying Tiger Line, the first cargo air carrier service in the United States, agreed to ship Orbis' medical supplies to international locations for free. Years later, when FedEx began negotiations to buy Flying Tiger, there was concern at Orbis that FedEx would not continue the gratis shipment of medical gear.

They were wrong. The shipping conglomerate was about to become a key Orbis benefactor.

Steve Charles, who had been building a reputation as a preeminent retinal surgeon in Memphis, lived in the same neighborhood as Fred W. Smith, the founder of FedEx, and the two had become casual friends. Charles was able to facilitate a meeting between Smith and Oliver Foot, who had become the executive director of Orbis.

The son of Jamaica's last British governor, Foot was also a former Shakespearean actor, lobbyist to the English parliament, cowboy, public relations executive, evangelist, preacher, and rock band manager. The central love of his professional life, however, was Orbis, and he unabashedly asked anyone for assistance for the charity.

Foot had contacted Charles with what he described as a double request. In addition to the meeting with Smith at FedEx, Foot asked for another favor: He knew Charles was a friend of then-U.S. Senator Al Gore. Orbis was trying to fly a mission into Moscow and needed political influence to obtain approval. Gore's father, who had also been a senator from Tennessee, was a close colleague and business associate of Armand Hammer, an American industrialist with numerous economic and political relationships within the Soviet Union. Charles made the introductions, and the Gores, father and son, used their connections to convince the U.S. State Department to approve the Orbis flight into Moscow.

Foot, meanwhile, came to Memphis to meet with Fred Smith and Charles to discuss the medical shipments he hoped would continue after FedEx completed its purchase of Flying Tiger. He and Ueltschi understood that any assistance from FedEx was an important imprimatur for the organization. The connection not only would advance Orbis' reputation and mission, but it would also generate other financial and corporate support.

When Charles and Foot met with Fred Smith, the doctor assumed the meeting would last an hour. Instead, it went only minutes beyond introductions.

Charles remembered, "Fred just told us, 'Sure, I know Orbis and Al Ueltschi, and I know of you, Mr. Foot. What does Orbis need?' We told him about the continued requirement for the shipment of medical supplies to countries being visited by Orbis. He said, 'Hold on,' picked up the phone, called someone, and told that person to continue helping Orbis after the Flying Tiger Line was purchased. He put the phone down and asked, 'What else do you need? FedEx will help. Just let us know what else you need.' We left so quickly we didn't even know if we'd done any good."

They had, of course, accomplished immense good.

As for the Orbis flight to Moscow, Charles was invited to join the team as the only retinal surgeon. It was 1987, and the DC-8's mission was no different than any other trip; doctors were to be presented middle-difficulty cases that demonstrated how to manage the patient's treatment. Physicians working with Orbis adhered to a list of guidelines for their international surgeries. The goal was always to "train the trainers," who could then spread knowledge and technical skills throughout the host country. Rules prevented physicians from operating on celebrities or patients who might exercise political or social pressure to receive care.

But sometimes exceptions are unavoidable.

The morning Charles joined the Orbis team in Moscow to begin looking at charts and examining patients, a group of Soviet armored personnel carriers approached the DC-8 sitting on the ramp at the airport. A large man with a flattop haircut, thick wire-brush eyebrows, and a big neck stepped out of the car and entered the plane. His drab, gray uniform was wallpapered with medals. Clearly a man of some importance, he was not, however, formally introduced to the doctors. He was guided to an exam chair by his translator, whom the doctors were confident was a KGB agent. A slit-lamp was pulled in front of the officer's eye, and Charles was handed a lens to conduct an examination.

The problem was obvious to the doctor.

"He has a piece of titanium embedded in his retina," Charles said to the translator. "It is sitting on an epimacular membrane, a kind of plate of scar tissue, and has caused a macular pucker. It is also in contact with vessels on the optic nerve."

The Russian translator did not appear to understand.

"This is a pretty straightforward case," Charles explained. "I can operate tomorrow and fix it. Should only take about 30 minutes."

This was translated for the two Russian retinal surgeons onboard the plane.

"*Nyet.*"

"*Nyet.*"

Charles looked at the translator. "Please tell them I can do it tomorrow, no problem."

After another exchange, the translator turned back to Charles. "They say is not possible."

"Please tell my colleagues that, yes, it is."

The Soviet general left with his small entourage and without any reaction to the news his vision might be saved in his eye. Perhaps he had no idea how precarious his eye condition actually was.

The next morning, the general arrived at the surgical facility where Charles was to conduct his retinal operations. TV cameras had been strategically located, and the surgery was obviously going to be recorded or broadcast.

"All I could think of," Charles later said, "was, man, if I blow this, I am headed to Siberia."

The surgery was broadcast over Russian national television to hospitals throughout the country so other physicians and surgeons could learn from the procedure. Charles, of course, did not bungle his operation, and the next day at a press conference with Pravda and Tass (the Soviet media networks) and 400 dignitaries, the taped surgery was played again. Ueltschi and Foot watched from the front row, confident in Charles' skills and sure that Orbis would be able to develop a deep and trusting relationship with the Soviet Union. No one, however, ever learned the name or the exact title of the general whose sight was saved by a man he had never met prior to his examination and whose name he probably never knew.

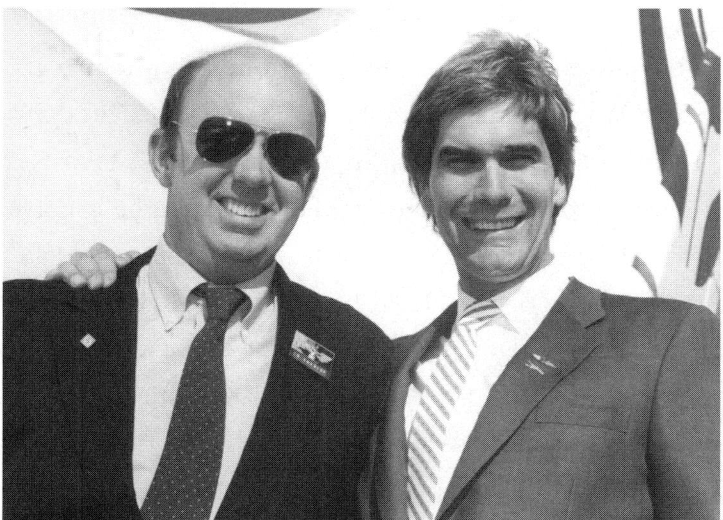

Charles and Oliver Foot in Moscow. Foot was instrumental in Orbis launch.

Back in the States, Orbis had been raising funds to buy a larger and faster aircraft to serve as the traveling hospital. The organization had found an affordable DC-10 jumbo jet and was considering its purchase. Fred Smith, continuing his commitment to Orbis, later sent Ron Wickens, his vice president for strategic projects, with Charles to Waco, Texas to examine the plane's mechanical viability and potential value as a flying eye hospital. Charles had become a licensed twin-engine jet pilot, and his mechanical inclinations had led the doctor to achieve substantial expertise in aircraft and avionics. The DC-10 was purchased, but the DC-8 kept flying for three more years as the jumbo jet was refurbished and retrofitted.

Charles continued his close association with Orbis. He turned to his friend Senator Gore for another diplomatic favor—to authorize travel to Cuba. Charles was aboard the DC-8 when it made its first trip to that communist country in 1991. When the external power system failed and the plane could not be started at the airport in Havana, the doctor's electrical engineering skills were essential in fixing the auxiliary power unit.

Upon completion of the extensive retrofit of Orbis' first DC-10, the aircraft was positioned in Hong Kong for its inaugural mission, a 1994 trip to Beijing. Charles, an accomplished jet pilot by then, with thousands of hours of airtime, flew in the right-hand seat of the aircraft for part of the trip. As the giant plane touched down, he noticed the old Orbis DC-8 hospital on public display at the airport, an acknowledgment by the Chinese of the valued assistance provided to the country by the charity. Charles later conducted the first retinal surgery aboard the new plane while in Beijing.

Each Orbis trip is the product of more than a year's effort of advance preparation, as the staff works to identify the right doctors and hospitals in the host country, even who will be allowed to scrub for surgery and who can take advantage of the education offered. The nonprofit medical service often leaves behind experts to sustain the improved practices and standards.

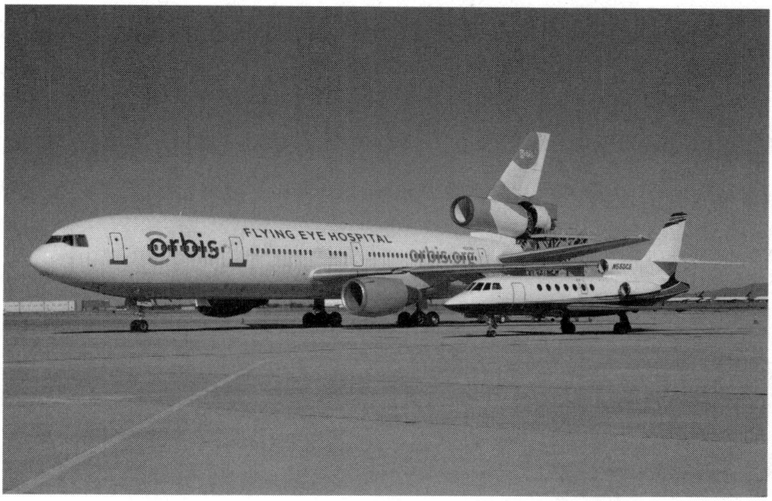

Orbis Flying Eye Hospital DC-10 next to Charles' Falcon 50 jet, Victorville, California

"Orbis is appreciated everywhere we go," said Charles. "But the Chinese seemed particularly grateful for our assistance. We were treated to a grand reception at the Great Hall of the People, and they understood that Orbis has nothing to do with politics. When we shake hands with politicians or great leaders, we make certain everyone understands this is not a U.S. project but an international effort. We don't do political things. We do surgery to teach surgical technique."

The mission of Orbis has only grown more ambitious with each passing year, and FedEx has been intimately involved for more than three decades. Not only did it donate the $2 million MD-10, it contributed another $5 million in cash and assistance, such as pilots' and mechanics' services. The third-generation Orbis airplane is the only non-land-based hospital in the world that is U.S. accredited by the AAAASFI (American Association for Accreditation of Ambulatory Surgery Facilities International) and is equipped with a state-of-the-art ophthalmic suite, treatment rooms, and a 46-seat classroom.

The interior design took advantage of FedEx's cargo expertise, is constructed of a series of nine custom modules that fit inside the cargo hull, and houses an IT and audio-visual center, a laser, pre-and postoperative examining spaces, a simulator and observation room, an administration office, a gold-standard operating room, substerile chambers, and a fully functional recovery room. The Flying Eye Hospital took six years and 250,000 man-hours to build, includes 17.6 miles of cabling, and contains 40 tons of medical equipment and a sufficient supply of teddy bears to provide one for every pediatric patient.

Orbis has become, however, more than a flying hospital. The plane and its people have become an airborne icon of man's humanity to man and how great movements can arise from small moments. Between 2011 and 2015, the organization facilitated, in various countries, the training of about 10,000 doctors and 104,000 nurses, biomedical engineers, and health-care workers. It provided 11.6 million eye screenings, and those numbers increase almost daily. There are about 400 medical expert volunteers, including some of the world's most accomplished ophthalmological surgeons from 30 different countries, who provide training to medical teams in their local facilities and onboard the aircraft.

An estimated four dollars of positive economic and social impact is realized for every dollar spent on blindness prevention, which makes eye health one of the most cost-effective interventions in medicine and a powerful tool in efforts to alleviate poverty.

Orbis is one of the most successful charities ever founded. The average gift from private individuals is $76, but corporations provide donations of money and in-kind contributions that total much, much more. Their brands and identities are an indication of the nonprofit's influence. Corporations like Alcon and L'Occitane and their foundations, as well as the Yeung Yee Charity Foundation and the Emperor Foundation all have sponsored significant funding for each of the rooms on the Flying Eye Hospital. A charter airline company in Tulsa, Omni International, donated parts and systems from a retired DC-10 to get the new Orbis jet into the air. Orbis also offered sponsorships and naming rights. For an appropriate gift, individuals or organizations can have a signature nameplate attached to a seat back.

The day before the public unveiling of the MD-10 Flying Eye Hospital, Charles gave me a tour of the onboard facilities. His enthusiasm was infectious as he went from the classroom in the forward cabin to the operating and recovery sections aft. Charles was as excited as a teenager who had just bought his first car.

"We can do everything on here," he said. "The volunteer faculty will do cataract surgery, glaucoma surgery, corneal transplants, and pediatric surgery, and, of course, I plan to be teaching vitreoretinal surgery."

In the operating room, a three-and-a-half-foot-tall machine had been secured to a bulkhead. I recognized the sleek profile and walked over to briefly examine it. Charles stood by the door, speaking with his old friend Jack McHale, the relentless visionary who had raised millions for Orbis. As I suspected, the machine at the bulkhead was an Alcon Constellation vitreoretinal operating platform. Charles had designed about 80 percent of its tools, systems, and precision functionalities for microsurgery on damaged retinas. Even without the doctor present, his contributions would change the lives of people around the world.

"Can we go up to the flight deck, Doc?" I asked.

He led me back through the cabin and up the steps to the cockpit. Charles did not hesitate. He went straight to the left-side seat, normally occupied by the pilot, and began talking about the plane's systems and controls with the FedEx mechanic working there. After a few questions from Charles, it was obvious that the doctor was as knowledgeable about airplanes as he was about retinal surgery. Charles has loved aviation since he was a boy looking at airplanes at the Oshkosh Air Show in Wisconsin, where he visited his Swedish grandfather during summers.

Charles also loves the flight deck of any airplane. The convergence of technology and systems excites his endless curiosity. The avionics of jet aircraft have multiple sensitivities and levels of importance that probably appeal to him in the same way as those inside the human eye. The practice of medicine and the art of flight have an equal hold on him. He has trouble ever turning off his interest in either subject.

"I've never known anyone with his intellectual capacity to learn just anything he's wanted to learn," said Buddy Dawsey, the doctor's longtime friend and co-pilot on Charles' personal Sabreliner jet. "If a light comes on when we are flying, he thinks in terms of the pin and the ohms and the wiring schematic. I think of what I need to do to prevent something from happening. We complement each other that way, I guess. He's a very technical person with a very analytical mind."

Dawsey is no casual observer of aviation. The Federal Aviation Administration honored him in 2013 with the Wright Brothers Master Pilot Award for 50 years of flight experience and for advancing aviation safety and professionalism. He taught Charles to fly in the mid-1980s and has sat in the co-pilot's seat on almost every flight the doctor pilots.

Charles was still thinking about the new Flying Eye Hospital a few days after the plane's Memphis christening. He had been planning for his next Orbis journey for months; the maiden flight of the new hospital plane was set for September 2016. It was destined for Shenyang, a city of about eight million people in the far northeast of China. Charles was scheduled to be a part of the three-week mission and would perform vitreoretinal surgeries while teaching and training Chinese colleagues on the latest techniques. It seemed, though, that he wanted, a more permanent connection to the big jet and Orbis' work.

Because he had flown in the right-hand seat on the original DC-10's first flight into China, perhaps Charles was hoping to someday co-pilot the new jet on one of its trips. Whatever the reason, he quietly informed the Orbis leadership that he would make a donation for naming rights to the co-pilot's seat. He wrote a $100,000 check to the charity for the small, engraved plate that would bear his name and a dedication he would write.

Charles is not given to dreamy reverie. He tends toward the pragmatic—making plans and executing them, designing, improving, and building. These characteristics undoubtedly made him a difficult fit for academia. He likes to do things, not write about or overanalyze them. He will try and fail and try again, until he succeeds. And never, ever quit.

"Keep going, full throttle," he said. "There's no other way to live."

THIRTEEN

The Helpful Hand

The idea occurred to Steve Charles during his last year of medical school. The engineering part of his mind was tackling a challenge for surgeons that was related to microsurgery. How, he wondered, can you magnify your vision 15 times and expect your hands to compensate when they move into the surgical field? How could that happen? There needed to be a method for scaling down motion, velocity, and force. Charles was convinced that if there were a technology to accomplish what he called dexterity enhancement—a tool for the hand analogous to what the microscope provides for the surgeon's vision—it would have great value in critical types of surgery.

"You realize very quickly," Charles explained, "that if you scale down position mechanically, without interposing electronics and software, it's just not going to work. But I started to consider the mechanical aspects of this, how to make it happen. I thought it could be very important for surgery, if it could be made effective and safe. I wrote a white paper on it and gave it to Dr. [Ed] Norton" of BPEI.

At the time, there was little mechanical assistance to human surgery. Charles understood the solution was almost certain to become a form of robotics. The notion of precise control of minute movements had a design appeal to him and a practicality that was unavoidably attractive. However, at BPEI he was part of a growing medical institution that was focused on transforming intraocular surgery, and he turned his inventive mind in that direction.

Nor were robotics a primary concern as Charles was launching his private practice in Memphis. But they became of increased interest to him when his father, tragically, was diagnosed with a brain tumor. Without technology to enhance mechanical-movement control for surgeons, there was little the doctors could do for Charles' father after his diagnosis. That led to a conversation between father and son about the need for precise surgical robotics.

"My dad literally said to me, 'You need to work with the neurosurgeons to help patients like me,'" Charles recalled. "And not that long after he died, I started having nightmares that I wasn't doing it. I thought that I had to do what he told me to do, even though microsurgery is unnatural: To magnify your vision and not enhance your dexterity makes no sense, and when you are working with a 10-micron precision, it just becomes totally incredible."

Charles was prompted by his father's passing to begin examining the complications of those issues. Was there a mechanical method for filtering hand tremors? How could you get a return of tactile information between a "slave and tool" and a surgeon "master" and improve the linkage between the tool and the surgeon's hand? The most likely approach was to engineer some system to scale down motion, force, and velocity. Any such construct, Charles concluded, would be most effective if the operator were in the same room and not working remotely, and if the system recognized the importance of force control, not just position.

There also needed to be "no-fly zones," a term Charles applied to tissue spaces where the instrument did not intrude, even if the surgeon consciously tried to cross those boundaries. These zones could be guided by advanced imaging like MRIs or CT scans or by known and mapped anatomical features. Accidental intrusion into healthy tissue was avoidable using these tactics. Heavy tools, such as drills, effectively would also become "weightless" when they were driven by the surgeon's slight touch on the handle that guided their movements.

The purpose of Charles' efforts in robotics was to improve outcomes for neuro, spine, ENT (ear, nose, throat), trans-oral, and orthopedic surgeries. He was not focused on eye surgery. Removing handheld instruments quickly from the eye—say, in the event of patient movement by tracking the instruments' motion—is less dangerous than having a robotic tool in the eye. A dexterity-enhancement system could only be used for the eye if the patient was under general anesthesia, and Charles primarily uses local anesthesia for his vitreoretinal patients. Computerized surgical instruments have made doctors and designers begin to contemplate various uses of robots for vitreoretinal surgery, however. These are considerably different than the successful laser "robots" that have redefined the treatment of the front of the eye with precise corneal corrections to improve vision.

As he began to think about the engineering of surgical robots, Charles was also increasing his skills as a pilot. Aviation had a practical appeal because his growing reputation as a leader in the vitreoretinal field meant additional travel demands. But aircraft functionality, design, and systems also intrigued him because of their engineering. The slightest touch on the trim-tab button altered the flight of an airplane, and those types of surface controls prompted the doctor to start thinking of their applications to surgery.

"I was in the cockpit," he said, "flying along, and I asked myself about what the autopilot does in the soft-flight mode. Really, it does the same thing I do as the pilot, but does it faster with almost no lag time. Humans can't do those things as fast. Autopilots have three orthogonal gyros to stabilize the rudder, elevators, and ailerons, which are analogous to the surgeon's three semicircular canals in the inner ear. This is when I first thought about the term 'dexterity enhancement' and scaling down the motion of a surgeon's hands. What it's about is scaling force, position, velocity, and acceleration, and if you filter the movement at 5 Hertz, you can remove a surgeon's hand tremor to improve microsurgery outcomes."

Charles might have been forgiven if he had chosen to ignore his curiosity regarding robotics engineering. He had other things on his plate: His practice in Memphis was growing rapidly with the spread of his reputation as a surgeon, and he was launching a company to design and build the next generation of vitreoretinal surgical tools. Nevertheless, Charles was hopeful his robotic concepts would improve other kinds of surgery. There were numerous reasons for his optimism.

Alan Morimoto, a young researcher at Sandia National Laboratories in Albuquerque, New Mexico, heard that Charles was working on developing surgical robots through a new company he'd founded, called MicroDexterity Systems. Morimoto had begun exploring similar projects, and he contacted the eye surgeon to see if he might be interested in a relationship with the national lab. Charles' work would be enhanced by the addition of other bright minds and, possibly, the resources of the federal government to promote and expedite research and development. MicroDexterity System eventually signed a cooperative research and development agreement (CRADA) with Sandia Labs.

Despite his many responsibilities, Charles managed to travel frequently to the New Mexico facility and lead the work on creating the surgical robots he envisioned. To make microsurgery safer and more effective, he wanted to incorporate the most effective haptic force feedback—the feedback provided by a surgeon's touch—into a manual, operate-by-wire system controlled by the surgeon. Tissue-information feedback was most likely to be conveyed in the 20–300 hertz range; less than 20 hertz would deliver no tissue information to the operator and would cause fatigue. Another goal was weightlessness of surgical tools that had precision approach and minute movements but did not affect side-to-side or reverse ranges of motion.

Building a robot in the 1980s to do microsurgery came with serious technological challenges. The computing power required called for huge mainframes and processing capacity that were not readily portable. As computers evolved, though, the hardware shrank, and moving the devices to surgical theaters and operating rooms became less problematic.

Eventually, Charles contacted one of the world's premier neurosurgeons, Robert Spetzler, M.D., of the Barrow Neurological Institute in Arizona. Spetzler's specialty was in cerebrovascular diseases and skull-based tumors, and he had the experience and skills to tell Charles if his early robotic efforts showed promise.

"He had defined a surgical robot that we evaluated," Spetzler said. "And we had it here in the laboratory. We also went up to New Mexico to see it, and it was a very clever piece of machinery with great feedback properties. I think it was way ahead of its time. Obviously, robots and surgery remain very much in a state of evolution. I think Steve's machine's ability to increase or decrease the movements, the actual amount of tactile feedback, was what separated it from the run-of-the-mill robots. I give him a lot of kudos for that. Steve is a very bright, triple-A personality."

The surgical robot was named MicroDex, but Steve had also begun additional designing around an already operational industrial robot called ParaDex, which was developed for assembly tasks. His robotic work had attracted the attention of NASA and the Jet Propulsion Laboratory (JPL) in Pasadena, and MicroDexterity Systems signed a technology cooperative agreement (TCA) with JPL. Soon, Charles was making multiple trips to California to work with NASA's engineers on a robot they identified as RAMS, or Robotic-Assisted Microsurgery. As JPL described it, "The RAMS workstation will enable new procedures of the brain, eye, ear, nose, throat, face, and hand."

NASA was overly optimistic about the commercialization of the evolving product at the close of the 1990s. JPL began to publicize the robot as a surgical system. And although it was not ready for use in the operating room, there were early plans to have it fly on one of the space shuttles as part of an experiment to cleave protein molecules in weightless environments.

The space agency's marketing language was clearly intended for a specific, narrow audience: "The RAMS not only refines the physical scale of state-of-the-art microsurgical procedures, but also enables more positive outcomes for average surgeons during typical procedures—e.g., the RAMS workstation controls include manual positioning and tracking in the face of myoclonic jerk and tremor that limit most surgeons' fine motion skills."

NASA's plans for the robotics were never fully executed, however. There is no record of the RAMS device traveling on a shuttle, and no medical applications materialized. None of that affected Charles' company. The doctor had hired a young engineer to work at InnoVision, and he discovered that Michael Stuart had a background in robotics from his days at the Massachusetts Institute of Technology (MIT). Stuart would play a role in the sale of the OCM to Alcon and would help wind down InnoVision.

Stuart later moved to Albuquerque, and when he called Charles about an eye problem, the doctor invited him out to visit the robotic labs at Sandia to see what was being built. A great deal of the work recalled ideas he and Charles had discussed a decade earlier. In fact, Stuart was still interested in the concept of surgical and industrial robotics. The meeting led to Stuart's being hired as the CEO of MicroDexterity Systems.

"I had done some work at MIT," Stuart said. "It was advanced training on robotics and intelligence, and when Steve learned that, he suggested it would be very nice if we could make the MicroDexterity robots do eye surgery. We first had these conversations back in the '80s, and if you look at that challenge from a technology standpoint in '87, those computers would've filled a small office. Fast forward 15 years or so. We met in Albuquerque, and we were putting these robots together using off-the-shelf, but high-powered industrial PCs. They had more power than the Cray supercomputers in the mid-'80s. Suddenly, in a manageable package the size of a shopping cart, we had technology we could go out and do medical procedures with."

The question became what *type* of surgeries were best suited to precision robotics. Charles thought that skull-based neurosurgery might be transformed by robots, but other opportunities appeared to be more viable. During the '90s, several manufacturers of medical devices were attempting to innovate new systems for cardiac surgery, and Charles decided to show his MicroDex robot to Ken Charhut of the Baxter Healthcare Corporation. Charhut was then the president of new business initiatives for Baxter's cardiovascular surgery division. He was looking for a product that would facilitate operations on the beating heart.

"That was kind of the 'out there' exercise that we were looking to see what we could do with," Charhut said. "One of the features of Steve's machine was its ability to track motion and be very precise. Heartport was coming out with its port-access product for cardiac surgery, and a company called CardioThoracic Systems was coming out with a beating-heart project that used surgeons' hands. Baxter didn't have a play in either at the time."

Baxter, under Charhut's leadership, invested in MicroDexterity and conducted a feasibility project for various types of cardiac surgery with the robot. The conclusion, according to Charhut, was that the technology "wasn't developed enough at the time" to accomplish the designated tasks. However, Charles asked Charhut to join the board of MicroDexterity, and Charhut recommended that they "point the robot in a different direction, because robotic cardiac surgery hadn't taken off." There were, he said, "easier clinical targets to play to."

Stuart had similar inclinations. California companies had solidly established a niche for heart devices, and, according to Stuart, there was "a good indication that because of interventional cardiology, cardiac surgery was a declining field." MicroDexterity's product line, therefore, was pivoted toward precision bone surgery. From a strictly business perspective, there was the potential for greater financial success: Launching the robot products into bone surgery offered more reimbursement than eye operations. And neurosurgery of the brain and spine were also good areas to focus on in order to make the company financially sound before developing other products.

Robert Spetzler, the renowned brain surgeon, saw much of the future of his discipline in the MicroDex robot when he brought it into his research operating room in Arizona.

"We used it to drill, for example, the skull," he said. "And that's where the haptic feedback was so remarkable. So, if you think about it, it's basically taking a heavy instrument, and instead of having your hand lifting that instrument, it suddenly becomes weightless, because you are only moving a joystick. You can ratchet it up and down, and you can use your dexterity in your hand. You can eliminate tremors in your hand. It is clearly the future for how we are going to be doing surgery."

Spetzler, in fact, was sufficiently impressed that he encouraged two other firms, Medtronic and later Stryker Corporation, a global provider of medical products, to go forward with MicroDexterity Systems, whose investors included Baxter, Allegiance Health, V Mueller, and Medtronic. An estimated 50 venture capital firms declined opportunities to put money into the business, but Charles and Stuart concentrated their efforts on bootstrapping the company to a positive cash flow, which is why there needed to be a strategy (like any start-up's) that pointed a direction to the shortest path to revenue, and that was neural and spine.

"We developed a variety of robots that could go in and do sculpting and hard-bone surgery," said Stuart. "The first doctors we worked with were neurosurgeons; it was a very viable area for us. But we moved from skull-based operations to spine surgery and dealt more and more with orthopedic doctors. We knew the company's bread and butter was going to be doing knees and hips."

The unfolding market plan led to a search for partnerships, in particular with medical-device manufacturers that had reputations of excellence and might be interested in investing. Charles and Stuart were thinking of contacting Stryker and asking for the use of an electrical bone saw to conduct a demonstration, when Stryker, which had heard of the MicroDexterity designs, got in touch with Charles about putting a bone saw on the end of a MicroDex robot. To see how that might work, Stryker sent an artificial bone with manufactured knee implant on top. MicroDexterity recorded a video of their robot sculpting the bone to improve fit of the implant.

"We sent that video to them, and they were out to our office in New Mexico in a week," Stuart said. "After that meeting and some phone conversations, Stryker was the only company we talked to. They bought a stake in the company, and we felt like they might eventually want to buy MicroDexterity and absorb it into their businesses."

MicroDexterity was on the verge of being hugely successful. One of the world's greatest neurosurgeons was an advocate for the enterprise, as was a global medical manufacturer. The company was going to market a device that ought to address a large, unmet need for doctors. The financial potential was great.

Everything was coming together for Charles. He had a thriving practice in Memphis, his name was on his specialty's top-selling surgical platform, he was piloting his jet to professional engagements where he was in constant demand, and he was about to transform a completely different type of surgical procedure with his latest innovation. His life, he would admit, was quite good.

And then, he heard that strange sound in his head.

He knew what it was—a kind of "huffing" or "swishing" caused by the sound of blood moving through the veins. The medical term was "bruit," which described the sound of turbulence as blood flowed against an obstruction. The disturbance is usually only present in the carotid and femoral arteries. Charles first heard it in his head in the middle of the night when he went to the bathroom. During a routine exam for a gallstone, he asked his doctor to scan his carotids, and a "significant blockage" was discovered in one of the arteries, which proved to be related to his earlier cervical fusion surgery, not atherosclerosis.

He immediately understood he was at great risk of a stroke. Fortunately, one of the preeminent neurosurgeons in America was his research collaborator, and Charles emailed Spetzler to request a consultation. The obstruction could not be ignored. Fortunately, there was no accumulation of plaque in the artery, and that helped reduce the danger of the operation and increase its simplicity. A week after emailing the brain surgeon, Charles flew his jet to Phoenix for the delicate operation.

"He had a procedure called an endarterectomy," Spetzler said. "It gets rid of the blockage in a vessel that goes to the brain. The risk, of course, is that you have a stroke, maybe just a small one, but once you have one, you can't take it back. Steve was, obviously, very eager to avoid that risk. His blockage was quite serious. There were chances of everything from a small stroke to a brain hemorrhage and even death."

But none of that occurred. Charles awoke after a night in the hospital, took out his IV line, put on a Band-Aid, went to the airport, and flew his plane home to Memphis with his co-pilot and close friend, Buddy Dawsey. Although Spetzler had told him to use moderation in his recovery, Charles was in the gym the next day, "lifting 10 percent less." That was his interpretation of moderation.

In an email to Spetzler, Charles pointed out that there was "no cognitive impairment," which the neurosurgeon responded to by telling the eye surgeon, "You're not the first person to note oxygen is good for the brain."

Oxygen was once more flowing unimpaired into Charles' brain, and that always meant more ideas. He couldn't wait to get started, either. He was convinced his work as an engineer, inventor, and vitreoretinal surgeon was about to have significant impact.

Again.

FOURTEEN

The Oculárist

The man stared intently at my healthy eye, noting fine details. I had thought, mistakenly, that he was a doctor. Instead, he was more of an artist, taking note of his subject to make the unfolding creation more real, maybe even perfect. Nothing about me had ever been perfect, and I was humorously entertaining the idea that something artificial could attain that level on my person.

"I look at a lot of things," he told me. "How veined your eye is, pinkness on the perimeter, just how much visible white there is. It's all important to me."

"And then you paint something very close to a duplicate?" I asked.

"Not an exact copy, but very close. I don't want there to be noticeable differences. But it obviously has to look real."

"Yeah, real would be good," I said. "Especially since it's not."

He laughed, not very heartily.

It had turned out that, by the time I made my pilgrimage to Memphis to see Steve Charles, it was too late. My retinal tissue was no longer viable. It had been detached from the back of the eye for long enough that, even if it flattened against the retina, it would not function. Most of what remained inside my right eye was tangled tissue.

Charles said my eye was inoperable. All he could offer was counsel on a cosmetic approach, along with the unsettling declaration, undoubtedly true, that I probably would not have been in my predicament had I been in his care. He warned me not to have the eye enucleated—surgically removed—because the muscles were still attached, and that was important for making a prosthesis track the movement of my good eye.

I was about to become the wearer of an artificial eye created by a creative artist known as an ocularist.

"There are some very talented people in this field," Charles had said. "In your case, they would make something that looks like a large contact lens that sits on the globe that remains in the socket. It has become an art, and the prosthetics look real. No one can tell the difference."

The ocularist I found, Craig Pataky, worked out of a small house in central Austin that had been turned into an office. Two people wearing eye patches similar to mine were in the small lobby when I entered. The man and woman exchanged nods with me, acknowledging, I thought, our sad little monocular confederacy. Thirty minutes later, I sat across from the man who would return my face to its previous appearance.

Pataky, who had spent 10,000 hours in apprenticeship to earn his professional qualification and added 750 credits of related study, told me he had been drawn to his profession because of artistic instincts and a freakish accident as a boy in El Paso.

"You know how when you are a kid, and you and your pals are doing something stupid?" he asked. "And your mom sees you and tells you to stop because you might put your eye out? That actually happened to me. I put my eye out. It was just a one in a million thing."

"So? What happened?"

He lifted my eyelid and shined a light into the socket as he finished the story. "We were playing with a BB gun, that's all. Shooting it around, up into the air, and we seemed so far apart from each other. I just remember turning in my friend's direction and getting hit in the eye by a BB."

"Nothing to be done?"

"No, this was the '80s," he said. "Ophthalmology wasn't nearly as advanced as it is now. Plus, I think there was just too much damage."

Three decades later, Pataky was now an esteemed member of the American Society of Ocularists (ASO). He sat on its education committee and the organization's board of directors. In addition to his credentials, I was also encouraged by the fullness of his personal life. He was drawn to endurance sports like running and cycling and enjoyed scuba diving and snow skiing. Pataky was married, had two sons, and did not appear to have been inhibited by his monocular vision in any way. I liked him almost immediately.

I was hopeful when I left the ocularist's office. And that was an emotion I had not experienced in a long while.

My struggle to maintain the sight in my right eye had turned into a waterfall of misfortune. Dr. D had detected the cataract in my lens, which was the result, I later found out, of the steroid drops I'd taken to hold down inflammation in my eye. He immediately scheduled me for surgery to have an artificial lens implanted.

At that point, I had already been through five retinal operations and was hopeful that with the new lens my vision would be clear. The cloudy cataract would be gone, and the retina might have reattached against the back of my eye. Unfortunately, the cataract specialist who looked into my eye noticed that the capsule—the tissue that encloses the lens and separates the front of the eye from the back—had become thick and scarred.

"Your ophthalmologist is going to want us to open up the capsule," he said.

"I'm not sure what you are telling me."

"Well, think of it as a kind of clear, elastic tissue that encloses your lens. It helps you focus the lens, but it can also get traumatized and create obstruction to light."

"Yeah? I'm getting traumatized. Did that cause it?"

The doctor was behind a scope that he had been using to examine my eye. He flashed a bright light at my pupil, but I could not perceive it in the bad eye. Plus, he was ignoring my great wit.

"So, what does 'open it up' mean, then?"

"I need to fire the laser into your eye. We basically just cut an X or a plus sign in the middle of the capsule, and it releases it into a series of flaps that are then out of the way of entering light."

"Will they just be flopping around in there?"

"No, the tissue curls back and firms up; it completely stays out of the way."

"It feels like my eye is getting blasted and cut and shot up with laser like a damned building getting sandblasted."

"Understand your concerns," he said.

The cataract operation a few days later seemed to take only minutes, and the procedure to blow out my lens capsule the next week was a quick pull on the laser trigger. I was eager to know what the cataract surgeon might see beyond the capsule after it had been opened.

"Can you tell anything?"

He swung a light into my pupil and waited no more than 10

seconds before responding with the bad news: "I'm afraid your retina is still detached."

"Good Christ."

"Do you want me to call your retina specialist and tell him you are on your way over?"

"I suppose. But he hasn't exactly had the answers."

I had been unrealistically hopeful, seduced, I think, by the beauty and the simplicity of replacing a human lens with an artificial version. Millions of people with cataracts clouding their views had been given clear eyes by surgical implantations of lenses that functioned, in many cases, even better than the optics delivered by their genetics.

Implanting a lens to replace nature's milky version has become almost a robotic procedure. Patients sit in a waiting room and are given a mild sedative to deliver relaxation. One by one, as each patient is taken into the operating theater, the empty chair is filled by another person. Although it might feel like assembly-line medicine, cataract operations are safe, effective, and profitable for physicians.

As for the procedure, a tiny incision is made at the edge of the cornea and the folded lens is effectively injected into the opening. Inside the capsule, or, if it has been removed, the front chamber of the eye, the lens unfolds and slides naturally into position. In a matter of minutes, you can look out through the new lens at, hopefully, a much clearer view of your surroundings.

Cataract surgery, however, had changed for me. I didn't yet realize that my retina was still detached; either that, or there remained a significant amount of blood in the back of the eye, and I simply did not see through the haze. I reasoned, though, that if the retina were attached after the surgeries, I might be able to at least perceive the blood, but my eye was black, and I perceived no light. Emotionally, I was devastated by the results.

As my wife was driving me home, I tried to divine positive outcomes for my prognosis. Nature had evolved humans and all creatures to have two eyes that added depth and dimension to our range of sight. Over the course of the three-plus years of operations, I tried to contemplate the contours of my monocular life and to imagine how I would adjust and function. I continued to think that my eye still might heal if the tissue were allowed to quiet down. I briefly refrained from seeking further surgical fixes. Eventually, though, I went back into the operating theater—a cumulative total of nine times—and resorted to more gas, silicone oil, and the intermittent wearing of eye patches. There's not much difference between determination and desperation when your eyesight is at stake.

I went to spring baseball practice one more time, wearing the eye patch, hoping for healing. Outside of the psychological discomfort of adjusting to a dramatically reduced field of vision, there was no immediate way for me to measure what I was losing until I got back on the diamond. Few things had been more beautiful to me in my life than a spinning baseball moving toward a batter or a fielder and the artistry of changing the ball's direction to affect the course of the game.

I took infield grounders one final time at first base and realized I would never again have confidence in my ability to catch the ball. Batting practice had become a similar struggle since the first time I had tried it with one eye. I convinced myself both skills could be picked up again if I devoted myself to the business of adjusting my vision and working like an 18-year-old rookie instead of a 60-year-old man. I suppose I will always be a sucker for baseball's spring renewal.

A part of me has never learned to stop trying, regardless of how absurd my goal. If both my eyes had stayed healthy, there could have been more baseball in my future. But a decent, monocular baseball player, at any age, would require an amount of time and commitment I needed to devote to other projects.

Of course, there was always the chance that being a one-eyed, geriatric baseball player was not as improbable as I believed. In one document that I had read while trying to understand monocular vision, I came across a 1992 statistic that the Federal Aviation Administration (FAA) had licensed, up to that point in its history, 218 first-class, 739 second-class, and 2,623 third-class medical certificates to pilots who had only one eye. My chances of ever sitting in the captain's chair of an A-380, however, seemed as remote as playing center field for the Houston Astros.

One of the vitreoretinal surgeons I turned to for a second opinion, prior to meeting Dr. Charles, had suggested that I might want to simply stop having surgeries. There had been five procedures on my eye by the time I reached his office after being referred by Dr. D. His advice was to let go, adjust to a new type of existence, and get on with my life instead of grasping at the tendrils of hope my retina might be healed. As sound as this recommendation was at that moment, surrender has always been difficult for me, and I felt a need to keep trying until there was no hope.

My quest finally had led me to Charles' office in Memphis. Meeting him and understanding his range of achievements was a revelation. But even he could not save the sight in my eye. The story of another of Charles' patients kept popping into my mind as a touchstone on how much worse things might have been.

Mark Mullen's story, which I had encountered while conducting my personal research for a way to save my sight, was impossible to forget. His right eye had been troubled from the time of his birth, and when his mother had finally taken him to Charles' office, she thought her son might get the treatment needed to grow up with relatively normal vision. Small blood vessels, however, were growing aggressively inside the boy's eye, leaking protein, creating what the doctors called exudative material that turned into scar tissue and destroyed eyesight.

Not even Steve Charles was able to deliver a cure for Mark Mullen's ailment.

"My mom took me to Dr. Charles' office one morning when he wasn't seeing patients," Mullen remembered. "He sat me down and started explaining things very plainly, the best he could to an eight-year-old, and did everything he could to make me feel comfortable. I knew my worst eye had to come out, but I thought he would do the operation. It turned out, though, that Chris Fleming, one of the best guys in the world for doing enucleation surgeries, was right down the road. Dr. Charles drove me there, gave the surgeon a full oral history, and then, I was okay with him doing the operation."

Mullen remembered telling his mother that his eye "felt a lot better out of my head than it did in my head." Charles also connected Mullen's family with an ocularist who created a custom artificial eye that tracked the movement of the boy's remaining eye. Over the next four years, the surviving eye provided stable, if minimal, vision to Mullen. However, the various treatments he was receiving for problems in the functioning eye led to cataracts.

Charles treated Mullen by using laser on the proliferating vessels and capillaries in his eye, and the boy's vision stabilized almost until he had finished high school. Then, it resumed deterioration. To stop the growth of blood vessels in the eye, Charles began a protocol of Avastin injections, a cancer drug that was being used off label. Mullen said any improvement in his vision as a result of the intraocular shots and IVs were not worth the ongoing pain and inconvenience. According to Mark, the doctor also tried him on another drug, Macugen, which he said, "kind of worked to improve my sight."

"I don't remember the timeline exactly," Mullen said, "but my iris in the remaining eye started bleeding with leaky capillaries. You know, you can put a drop of blood into a bucket of water and make it hard to see through. Dr. Charles sent me to an oncologist, and I did six weeks of an IV of Avastin every day. That frond of capillaries in my iris went away, and my tumor calmed down. I remember it had only been approved for colorectal cancers, and I heard one of the nurses say, 'How'd they fix his eye with that ass-cancer drug? Did you see he just got up and walked to the bathroom? He can see.'"

For seven years, Mullen struggled through a master's degree program in social science at Murfreesboro State University, but his vision was constrained by what he described as "looking through a lava lamp, and an amorphous, greenish haze full of blurry shit that moves around in some colors."

As he approached the age of 40, Mullen was facing even more difficult choices. His left eye was worsening with more than 30 years of accumulated scar tissue on the retina, a mostly nonfunctional iris, no useful lens in the eye, and all vitreous previously removed for surgery.

"The eye looks horrible, just nasty ugly, and it barely opens," he said. "I call this my five-martini eye. People think my prosthetic is the good eye. I suppose I was lucky to have functional vision for the vast majority of my life—six years functionally blind but 32 years with some kind of useful sight. I also think that if I had not been in Dr. Charles' care that I would have been blind in both eyes very early in my life. He tacked on 20 years of vision I would not have had without him."

What caused Mullen's eyes to fill with blood vessels and subsequent scar tissue? No one has ever ventured a likely explanation of the pathogenesis of his problem, and Mark still wishes for a full genome test because he believes that somewhere in the VEGF signaling cascade, he has a mutation. His own diagnosis is that endothelial cells are producing too much VEGF or oversensitive receptors. However, Charles examined three generations of Mullen's family on both the maternal and paternal sides and found nothing more than cataracts.

"It's just capillaries where they're not supposed to be," Mullen said.

The precise cause is a mystery that Mullen will live with. At the end of his fourth decade, he decided there was too much pain and frustration in dealing with the remaining eye for only a slight registration of light and shadow. Mark went to Charles and told him he planned to have the remaining eye removed. The doctor, who had seen Mullen suffering without cure for his entire life, understood the decision to choose complete darkness over pain and slim hope.

"Mark is a very brave young man," Charles said.

And I knew that I was not. I was scared.

People tend to fear blindness, the complete loss of any vision, more than just about everything in life. The emotional response and adjustments of the sighted who end up blind are undoubtedly different than those who began life without vision. But there are commonalities in the challenges to living without seeing. A research study published by *JAMA Ophthalmology* in 2016 indicated that 88 percent of more than 2,000 online respondents said that good vision was vital to their overall health. They ranked losing vision as equal to or worse than a loss of hearing, memory, speech, or even a limb, probably because, according to 47 percent of those interviewed, it would have the most effect on their daily lives. A little over half of those surveyed were aware of various diseases and conditions of the eye, but a quarter said they had no idea of any of those issues, and only half knew that smoking put eyesight at risk.

There is a clinical term for the fear of blindness: scotomaphobia, which comes from the Greek word *scotomas*, meaning blindness. This phobia tends to result from medical conditions like glaucoma, cataracts, or retinal detachments, but the fear can develop in people without any of those problems. Bright lights might cause a visual sensitivity, and scotomaphobia can evolve from such experiences. The condition often causes people to overschedule regular optical exams and to even contemplate diseases they might get that could lead to blindness.

I was afraid, and I had none of the reserves of courage that Mullen used to deal with his condition. I may not have been a scotomaphobe yet, but fear was creeping up on me. What if my other eye went bad? Despite that possibility, I always was able to turn my mind away from that outcome. My free time without visual problems was spent playing hardball, riding mountain bikes and motorcycles, reading endlessly, writing, and staring at starlit skies in the Texas Trans-Pecos. The notion I might lose some of that if my vision did not recover kept me restless and worried, but my greatest apprehension was not being able to make a living to take care of my family.

The time to move on had arrived. So here I was, in Craig Pataky's office for one of my final visits.

The ocularist inserted a soft, prosthetic form that had been used to make an anatomically correct acrylic fit at an earlier visit. Pataky took out a small brush with fine hairs and began to mark specific points of reference on the insert while I stared blankly out his window at the Texas sun.

"I suppose you've never had anyone paint on your eye before," he said.

"Uh, not so much, no."

He stared at my healthy eye as intently as any artist contemplating his subject and began to paint pink veins and the brown striations of an iris onto my prosthesis. In the end, there was really no way an average observer would realize they were looking at something artificial. No one other than myself and my doctor was ever going to see the shrunken, convoluted, grayish walnut of a globe resting in the socket on the right side of my head. I even ask my wife to not enter the bathroom when I am taking out the scleral shell for cleaning. As long as I am wearing it, which is constantly, I look as normal as the guy next to me.

There was a process of adjustment, though. I was always cautious on my motorcycle and slowed even for green-lighted intersections, but riding with one eye, I tended to keep my head moving from left to right to regain a field of vision I had lost. I had no uncertainty or fear while riding at highway speeds. I have done multiple trips of thousands of miles, including a 1,600-mile weekend to chase the total solar eclipse from Texas to Nebraska. Rebuilding my consulting practice was tedious and time consuming, but clients resumed calling for projects, and my task queue filled up with profitable and interesting technology assignments. Even though I was burdened with medical debt, I was convinced I could retire it with consistent employment over the next several years.

There was nothing forced about my positive outlook. Relief was an honest emotion after so much time and money spent dealing with an intractable health problem. The only thing I wanted more than my eyesight was to put this crisis in my past and resume my productive and fulfilling life. I had an abundance of friends, a wonderful wife and daughter, a distance runner's heart, bicycles and motorcycles, books and airplane tickets, and challenging projects that needed my insight and experience.

But I slowly began to worry about my good eye.

FIFTEEN

Miracles and Medicine

The diminutive woman sat quietly, comfortably dressed for a visit to the doctor's office. In the back hallway that gave Steve Charles private access to his patients, his assistant Sabrina Newsom told him the patient's name and briefly reminded him of the issues with the eyes he was about to examine for the second time. Charles entered the room, offered a quick hello, and turned to study a scan on the computer screen before looking back at his patient's expectant face.

"Well, I think I've explained this before," he said, "but your eyesight will continue to deteriorate without appropriate treatment, and laser is just no longer the best approach for diabetic retinopathy."

"So, you're saying the shots then?" she asked. "Right into my eye?"

"Yes, we put a topical anesthetic on the surface of your eye so you don't really feel much in the way of discomfort."

"But I thought the laser used to stop the bleeding?"

"It can, but new abnormal blood vessels grow, and there's scar tissue. That can reduce your vision as well. The drug we use for the shots not only stops the growth of new leaky capillaries but also gets rid of the others. It doesn't just stabilize your vision where it is, it improves it. Many people get back to near normal."

The woman sighed softly and leaned forward, resting her elbows on her knees. She appeared to be near 60 and had been struggling with the concept of a needle entering her eye even as her vision deteriorated from macular edema caused by diabetes.

"Okay, then, that's what I'll do."

"That's the best," Charles said. "We'll have you in once a month for an injection, and you'll be amazed at how well the treatment works. Most people are. And no side effects to worry about, either. We'll get you up front right away to get your first injection today."

The doctor rose, went back into the interior hallway, and looked at his phone briefly before telling me about the drug that was about to be placed in his patient's eyes.

"These drugs, they're called anti-VEGF"—for Vascular Endothelial Growth Factor—"and they are nothing short of miraculous," he said. "They effectively end the new blood vessel growth in the diabetic eye or for anyone dealing with wet macular degeneration. The bleeding in the eye stops, the new vessels regress, and your eyesight is saved. Frequently, it's returned to near what it was before. We know of almost no reactions. The only treatment in the past was to put in laser to stop the bleeding, but there was often scar tissue that had to be removed. And those operations tended to lead to other complications like cataracts and glaucoma."

Three decades earlier, Steve Charles had been in Israel to honor the researcher whose work had led to the treatments he had just offered. Isaac Michaelson had postulated that there was a molecule the human body dispatched to grow blood vessels in parts of the anatomy that were oxygen deprived. These chemical signals and the process to prompt the formation of new blood vessels is known as angiogenesis and includes migration, growth, and differentiation of endothelial cells that line the inside wall of blood vessels.

Controlling that biological process now offers great hope for cancer treatments and patients losing their eyesight through wet macular degeneration, diabetic macular edema, proliferative diabetic retinopathy, and retinal vein occlusions.

The story of the discovery of VEGF and the medical advancement to control its effects offers an object lesson in the value of both government and private research and their combined benefits to humanity. Michaelson first described the signaling peptide as what became known, initially, as the Vascular Permeability Factor (VPF), and proving its existence was also a part of Steve Charles' original charter when he was appointed to the National Eye Institute (NEI) of the National Institutes of Health (NIH) when he left BPEI in Miami during the seventies. In an early experiment, he had injected vitreous of a diabetic patient into the eye of a rhesus monkey, and it developed neovascularization, which effectively satisfied Michaelson's postulate for the existence of VPF, later more accurately described as Vascular Endothelial Growth Factor, or VEGF. A skeptical NEI pathologist kept a report from being published because it was not based on pathological confirmation.

The endothelium is a single-cell layer that lines the inside of every blood and lymphatic vessel in the human body. Endothelial cells have unique and critical functions in blood vessels as small as capillaries. These include fluid filtration, hemostasis, hormone trafficking, and even the tone of the blood vessel itself. They are also responsible for angiogenesis.

While medical science understood most of the role of endothelial cells, the notion that they might send a biologic message to parts of the body to prompt the growth of new veins seemed, at best, theoretical if not improbable and maybe impossible to prove, until the work of a postdoctoral student at the University of California,

San Francisco (USCF). Dr. Napoleone Ferrara, who had a background in reproductive endocrinology, made an intriguing discovery while examining pituitary cells. One of his experiments indicated that certain cells in the pituitary gland produced various factors that were capable of inducing endothelial cell growth. Fascinated, Ferrara began a second post doctorate in biochemistry to try to isolate what was later known as VEGF.

Isolating VEGF had the potential for dramatic medical implications. If the body signaled its own neovascularization, identifying how that happened meant the process of angiogenesis might be medically controlled. Medicine could possibly be designed to restrict vascularization in regions that are harmed by natural angiogenesis. To accomplish this, an antibody needed to be developed. Diabetics, for one example, tend to lose their central vision in the macula as a result of capillaries that leak and create macular edema, a swelling in the tissue that delivers the most important part of the visual field. There also might be the ability to use an anti-VEGF molecule to control tumor development by starving them of blood and oxygen.

In 1988, Ferrara decided to leave UCSF and join the pharmaceutical giant Genentech to do research on reproductive drugs. Although that work did not produce commercial results, the company afforded its scientists time to pursue their personal areas of interest. Ferrara followed his curiosity back to looking for VEGF. Similar research was being conducted at Harvard Medical School by M. Judah Folkman, M.D., who had founded the field of angiogenesis in an attempt to stop the growth of tumors.

"First, we attempted to isolate and characterize VEGF," Ferrara said, "which took us several years. We began with the basic science such as isolating, sequencing, cloning, and characterizing VEGF.

It was a very exciting time. Then, we needed to convince ourselves that this was something worth testing in humans. Genentech is a great place to do research. It has wonderful facilities and technology, which allowed us to answer some of these questions. After years of work, we developed the humanized antibody, Avastin (bevacizumab), which entered the clinic in 1997."

Even Ferrara seemed surprised at the potential of his findings.

"At that time," he said, "it would have been difficult to predict it, but VEGF proved to be a fundamental molecule in vascular development and in angiogenic processes in the adult. It became clear that it plays a key role in embryonic development. Also, VEGF appears important in skeletal and reproductive angiogenesis. However, the most significant biomedical implications of VEGF concern its role as a mediator of pathological angiogenesis, such as that associated with cancer and intraocular neovascular disorders."

The drug's early clinical success was the result of focusing research on blood vessels providing nutrient oxygen to cancer tumors. Avastin quickly became essential to a standard treatment for a variety of cancers, particularly those of the colon. Depriving cancer of blood reduced the associated risks of metastasis. Cancer patients tended to live longer when treated with Avastin, but the drug's *curative* rates were much lower than anticipated.

Ferrara continued his research on the cloning of anti-VEGF antibodies and soon co-discovered the role of VEGF in retinal disease. Specifically, he had been looking at how an angiogenesis inhibitor might help the problem of age-related macular degeneration (AMD), which affects tens of millions of people globally. Wet macular degeneration, caused by the proliferative growth of arterioles and capillaries under the retina, occurs in about one in five people with AMD. The vast majority instead suffer from dry macular degeneration, a deterioration of the central vision caused by the death of critical retinal tissue, the retinal pigment epithelium (RPE).

Ferrara's lab at Genentech isolated and developed the monoclonal antibody ranibizumab, which became known as Lucentis and began to be widely used as a first-line therapy to treat wet AMD. The drug was wildly successful in saving and even restoring eyesight and treating additional disorders like diabetic retinopathy, retinopathy of prematurity (a cause of blindness in premature babies), and retinal vein occlusions.

Monthly shots of Lucentis directly into the eye suppressed leaky blood vessels in the retina; a consistent protocol of injections generally allowed patients to gain back a great deal of their lost vision. The effectiveness of Lucentis quickly turned it into a $3 billion-dollar global product for Genentech.

A business problem arose, however.

The lead clinical researcher on Lucentis, Phil Rosenfeld, M.D., was an ophthalmologist at BPEI. Because he was the first author on publications that described the Phase I, II, and III clinical trials for Lucentis, he acquired great familiarity with its molecular structure and wrote about the drug in the October 2006 issue of the prestigious *New England Journal of Medicine.* Rosenfeld realized that the chemical design of Lucentis made it very similar to Avastin, which had been approved and was being used for the treatment of solid-growth tumors.

That prompted him to experiment.

"Rosenfeld tried Avastin on some of his patients with wet macular degeneration," said Jerry Helzner, who writes about the retina for numerous medical publications. "That's the kicker. He used it off label and without approval, took a big chance, and it worked. His patients started recovering their eyesight. This really caused problems for Genentech, because Avastin was cheap, at usually 50 bucks a shot. Lucentis was in the market at around $1,900 per injection. Genentech was competing with itself between those two drugs."

The cost, efficacy, and use of Avastin, Lucentis, and a later drug branded as Eylea (aflibercept) by Regeneron have generated controversy for doctors and Medicare and Medicaid health-care providers. Because macular degeneration affects the over-60 age group, the number of baby boomers with the problem has tended to put stress on the budgets of those government-supported health-care programs.

Eylea, which was designed to give patients up to eight weeks between treatments, did not appear to reduce expenses; the drug's manufacturer began reporting multi-billion-dollar revenue streams from their product.

But the 50-dollar charge for Avastin is the only one accepted by Medicaid, which means doctors treating lower-income patients for wet macular degeneration are compelled to use the drug off label. Roche, the company that owns Genentech, has historically refused to run Avastin through the long and costly process of FDA approval for wet macular degeneration. The firm insists Lucentis is the stronger and better therapy to end the intraocular growth of blood vessels that leak and cause blindness.

Meanwhile, a 2015 National Institutes of Health study indicated that using a less-expensive injection like Avastin had the potential to save Medicare $18 billion over a 10-year period.

Doctors like Charles point out there is a clinical difference between Avastin and the more expensive drugs, especially with regard to treatment of certain types of patients.

He said, "There are numerous doctors—and, really, this just irritates me to no end—who ask the question about which anti-VEGF do you use, as if it is a consideration of cost and not the patient.

Diabetic retinopathy patients have about 5,000 times more VEGF in their eyes than people dealing with wet AMD. Lucentis has 25 times higher molecular affinity for VEGF than Avastin. Proving a drug is good in wet macular degeneration is not the same as proving it works just as well for diabetic macular edema. People need their doctor to prescribe the *best* drug to be cured. It's that simple."

The patients in the waiting rooms of the Charles Retina Institute are not seeking an inexpensive solution. They want to see, and cost is only relevant in the context of third-party payers. There is probably no price that is too high for a person seeking to save his or her eyesight, even if it means spending down personal savings or burning up retirement funds.

Pharmaceutical companies that bring advanced drugs to the marketplace often invest hundreds of millions of dollars to develop their products. In a capitalist economy, they are not likely to be begrudged their profits, especially since government institutions tend to regulate more than innovate. To be sure, there are the inevitable profiteers; oncologists have been criticized for dramatic markups on Avastin and have been accused of "killing the goose that laid the golden egg."

"I have defended for-profit pharma," said Charles. "They cloned VEGF; physicians and universities didn't do it. Their years of work and research identified VEGF, and then, they made the antibodies. They also spent a ton of money and finally got it approved. Remember, prior to this, the standard of care for wet macular degeneration was laser. Only 5 percent of patients were eligible for that, depending on their conditions, and there was about a 50 percent success rate. We were also using steroids, which caused glaucoma."

None of those pharmaceutical companies have, however, conquered dry macular degeneration. The causes can be isolated, but addressing them has been a scientific challenge. Research indicates that dry macular degeneration is a product of genetics and is often exacerbated by smoking, a 350% to 500% increased progression risk for smokers. Eating a diet of leafy green vegetables can reduce risk by up to 25 percent, but the disease still occurs in some genetic groups. Hopes of gene therapy were dramatically reduced when a University of Iowa study showed the disease was polygenic, controlled by more than one gene. A drug to alter a single genome might have been worth pursuing, but a therapy that treats a random set of genes in each individual becomes a daunting, perhaps impossible, project, though research persists. There is also the biological problem of dealing with the immune system's multiple triggers, called the alternate complement pathway. These vary in each individual and can cause problems like inflammation or other acute issues in the retina.

Generally, several clinical studies are under way at any given time to find a cure for dry macular degeneration. Genentech has developed lampalizumab, a "monoclonal antibody fragment that inhibits complement factor D" (CFD) described as a "rate limiting enzyme involved in the activation of the alternative complement pathway." A Phase II study showed the anti-factor D treatment delivered a 20 percent reduction in the progression of lesions in geographic atrophy, meaning it stopped dying rods and cones from spreading. Phase III, though, did not justify further research and development, and Genentech stopped work on anti-factor D drugs when it announced "the primary end point had not been met."

Meanwhile, Apellis, a well-funded pharmaceutical research and development company, has reported an intravitreal drug (one injected into the vitreous) that reduces by 29 percent the advancement of geographic atrophy (dry AMD) when compared to a sham treatment. Those results, tallied over a 12-month period, were based on monthly injections. Published figures reported the second six months showed even greater progress by reducing geographic atrophy by 47 percent compared to the sham therapy. The higher figure might hint there is a more valuable, cumulative effect of the drug when administered over time. Company executives said they were very excited and planned to quickly launch Phase III studies.

The failure of pharmaceutical approaches continues to drive stem-cell-derived RPE cells and associated surgical approaches to treating dry macular degeneration. Stem-cell treatments seem as hopeful to many scientists as various drug studies. A National Eye Institute (NEI) project has spent years establishing protocols for developing useful cells and a mechanical technique for surgically inserting them into pigs. They also have created a methodology that solved moral and ethical concerns while providing the biological material needed for developing into healthy RPE cells. The FDA had to approve NEI's ethical practices for techniques to develop cells for humans and for deciding who donates and how the cells are used. Then, those processes had to be tested on the pigs used in research.

The federal government's attempt to cure dry macular degeneration with stem-cell surgery has been led by Kapil Bharti, Ph.D., and Juan Amaral, M.D., a soft-spoken and thoughtful Peruvian immigrant and vitreoretinal surgeon. The goal is to develop an autologous cell therapy (in which cells are obtained from the individual who will receive them as treatment) to avoid rejection by the recipient's eye. Doctors will obtain blood from the patient and transform induced pluripotent stem cells—which have an ability to develop into almost any type of cell in the body—into authentic RPE cells. These changed cells are then seeded onto a biodegradable scaffold and surgically placed beneath the retina, adjacent to the affected area of dying retinal tissue.

"We don't even know if this is going to work," Amaral said. "This is just the first stage. If we succeed, we'll file with the FDA to begin human clinical trials. But our surgical model starting out is with pigs. One of the reasons is that their eye is very similar to ours. Even though they don't have a macula, they have a central area in their eyes called the visual streak, and it has cones and is similar to our macula."

The process can be overwhelming. The autologous cells must be examined not just under an electron microscope but also with many other techniques to make sure that they support the visual cycle of the macula, that they properly pump nutrients, that they recycle visual pigment, and that they make VEGF at their basal end. The risk of rejection exists in both humans and animals.

An even more ambitious goal is to generate rods and cones, the photoreceptor cells themselves, and not just the RPE that keep them alive and functioning. This area of research and medicine is known as regenerative medicine. The purpose is to develop cell lines that can be used to study disease in the lab; disease in a cup. A more ambitious goal is to replace cells for diseases like age-related dry macular degeneration or retinitis pigmentosa. This approach is similar to what has been used in the early development of the NEI porcine study involving Steve Charles. Human cells are derived from a patient's blood or skin and can be induced to differentiate themselves into any cell type in the human body.

Biotech executive Carter Cliff has been involved in several pharmaceutical company start-ups focusing on therapeutic cell development. His latest effort is to grow cell lines that replace the dying photoreceptors in the retina.

"I think researchers see dry macular degeneration as an intractable problem for a pharmaceutical product," he said. "It seems an appropriate time to advance a new therapeutic approach. Specifically, you need to replace the RPE cells in the case of dry AMD, and, more generally, you need a photoreceptor. If it could be delivered early, you'd prevent the visual loss in an earlier-stage patient. Our whole approach is to reach the point where we can regenerate the photoreceptor that needs repair, and we are developing photoreceptors for transplant."

Cliff acknowledged the induced pluripotential stem cell study to create photoreceptor cells was at a much earlier stage than the NEI's project to develop and insert RPE cells. But he believes his nascent company's research will answer FDA questions sufficiently to be cleared, eventually, for human clinical trials.

Surgical protocols are challenging, regardless of the cells being placed into the eye. In the case of the NEI pig project, a laser must first be used on the animal's retina to kill RPE cells in a manner that mimics geographic atrophy in humans. The pig's macula has to be detached by injecting saline, which provides space between the choroid and the retina. An incision is then made into the eye so the scaffold of autologous RPE cells derived from stem cells can be inserted beneath the retina. In humans, this would be the time when the cells replace the RPE cells that have started to falter and reduce vision. The entire operation initially required about four hours.

Amaral, who had been to Memphis to observe Charles' work in 1999, inquired whether the eye surgeon might be interested in the RPE project. Charles suggested he would have *begged* to take part had he not been invited by Amaral. He began to visit the NEI and offered suggestions for improving surgical techniques.

Charles has considered his contributions to the research to be "minor," but according to Amaral, he's added "immense credibility" to the project. He has also shortened the operating time from 4 hours to about 25 minutes.

"Part of that was by eliminating the laser or diathermy to cauterize the retinal incision required for scaffold insertion," Charles said. "Both of those techniques cause retinal and RPE damage, visual field defects like scotomas, and the scarring of proliferative vitreoretinopathy. I also developed a spring-loaded wound clamp that works like an inverse speculum and holds in place the 2-plus-millimeter incision for scaffold insertion. This prevents loss of pressure in the eye with the large wound needed to insert the cells scaffold."

The operations with pigs also require that doctors use laser to destroy RPE in the animals, and for that they need anesthesia. Charles designed a device that eliminates both the laser and the anesthesia. He also developed a contoured, shorter, and lightweight handle to enhance the dexterity of the scaffold-insertion tool. Charles worked with Amaral's team on the insertion cannula design and, after a few operations, began outlining details and procedures to move the operation to human clinical trials. This will be of major importance; the number of people suffering from some form of age-related macular degeneration is estimated at 196 million worldwide by the year 2020 and 288 million by 2040.

Ultimately, if Bharti, Amaral, Charles, and the NEI team of physicians and researchers meet all the rigorous FDA standards for treatment, they will likely develop a bank for human RPE cells. Much depends upon whether the induced tissue responds and grows in the retina and creates RPE cells that can provide the metabolic support needed for the photoreceptors to keep them from dying. Even if photoreceptor cells can be grown using induced somatic cells, there will be a need for the underlying RPE. If the science and the results unfold as envisioned for the NEI model study, it will be followed by the initial surgeries in the human clinical trial.

And Charles is expected to perform the first operation.

SIXTEEN

Germantown

"Dad, I can't see out of half of my eye."

Carl Daniel was puzzled. He looked at his 14-year-old son and wondered if the boy was simply goofing around.

"Which eye, boy?"

"This one." Detorrius Daniel pointed at his face. "I'm scared."

"You see something, don't you?"

"Yes, but only halfway. Everything else is gone."

"I don't understand, Detorrius. You see me right now?"

"Yes, sir, but only half of your face."

"Okay, let's call the eye doctor. Might have to go to the emergency room."

Daniel quickly got his son to an optometrist, who told him Detorrius needed immediate treatment. Fortunately, Daniel had chosen a professional whose office was in the same building as that of Steve Charles. Detorrius and his father were sent downstairs to be examined by Dr. Stephen Huddleston, a fellow in the Charles Retina Institute, who was working alone while Charles was traveling.

"This poor kid's retina had just folded over like a taco," Huddleston explained. "This was a giant break, and I was here by myself. Dr. Charles' partner, Jorge [Calzada], was in London. I knew if this wasn't fixed right that the kid was going to go blind. I didn't have that level of experience, so I called up Dr. Charles. Blindness is simply not acceptable."

Charles and Buddy Dawsey had flown the doctor's personal jet to Philadelphia for a retina conference at the Wills Eye Institute.

Charles' response was quick. "Get him ready for surgery," he told Huddleston on the phone. "Buddy and I will head back to the airport and get the plane ready to fly back to Memphis tonight."

Huddleston, as smart as he is earnest, had made a critical decision that changed the life of Detorrius Daniel. The young doctor estimated that his own abilities only gave the Memphis teenager a 5 percent chance of having his vision restored. Charles would raise those odds of success to 95 percent.

"You want me with the coin-flip chance of success at best, or Charles with the good long odds?" Huddleston asked, when recounting the story. "I worried the entire retina might come loose, turn into a tissue ball, and not be fixable. A teenager would go blind. I talked to Dr. Charles again as he was getting his plane ready, and we both agreed this was the best decision."

There were, however, things that Charles didn't mention that night or any other time. As much as the aircraft had become an essential tool for his work, the operational costs would appear absurd to an uninformed observer. Fuel, maintenance, insurance, landing and hangar fees, and the inspections attendant to operating a twin-engine jet in American airspace put the hourly operating costs at about $5,200. The approximate two-hour trip from Philadelphia to Memphis with a return flight to rejoin the conference was almost certain to total more than $20,000. No patient or insurance company could be expected to pay the freight on such a trip. Charles quietly absorbed the bill for his emergency transportation.

"He did another thing that I think you should know about," Carl Daniel said. "I know he didn't tell you about this, because I know the kind of man he is. I was going through financial problems just then, and I had no idea how I was going to pay for these surgeries. He told me he would waive his bills. He didn't have to do that."

For Detorrius Daniel, the giant retinal break would have been a sentence to blindness before the development of new surgical techniques pioneered by Charles. Instead, the eye doctor spent just 45 minutes doing a surgical repair and then went back to the airport for his return flight to Philadelphia.

He had used laser to reattach the retina after he had removed the vitreous from the eye using the Constellation platform. A high-specific-gravity liquid, perfluoron (PFO), was infused into the eye to flatten the retina to the back of the boy's eye, and endolaser was applied. In two weeks, the PFO was removed, the retina remained attached, and the boy's vision was returned to previous levels of acuity.

Genetically, there are small population groups that are more predisposed to retinal detachment based upon extreme eye length and even factors like thinness of the retinal lining in the intraocular space. During a follow-up exam, Charles discovered that Detorrius' other eye was also showing retinal detachment. He made a similar surgical repair, and vision was again restored. The boy's genetic misfortune had been offset by the fact that he was born and raised in Memphis, saw an optometrist able to immediately refer him to Charles, and lived in an era when procedures like vitrectomy and laser reattachment had become almost routine.

"It's important to understand that, 30 years ago, he would have just gone blind," Huddleston said. "Giant breaks used to be absolute failures. Now, we are doing vitrectomies and using PFO, and there are 90 percent positive outcomes. I came to know the Daniel family very well. They understand their good luck and how bad things might have gone for their son."

"I am grateful this man came into our lives," Carl Daniel said. "He gave our son the opportunity to be successful. He has been able to see to get through school. My boy's funny, too. I guess he can see better than we thought. He thinks he's a ladies' man, and from what I can see, the girls seem to like him. He's a laid-back young guy who doesn't commit to a thing. Least not yet."

Stories like the Daniels' abound in Charles' life. He has often said that money is not a goal; it is what makes it possible to help people and do his research and inventing. Perhaps that accounts for the doctor's apparent ambivalence about being in business. Money is not a measurement of success for him, and he can be quite casual about it. None of his colleagues was surprised by a story of him taking a wad of hundred dollar bills out of his pocket and handing $3,000 to an Alabama nurse whose husband had left her and their kids without a way to pay the bills.

Judy Perry, who manages the finances of the Charles Retina Institute, said the doctor's kindness can be financially mystifying. "Sometimes," she said, "he is too good for his own good. If a patient is sitting there and has hard times and can't pay their bills, I've seen him pull money out of his pocket and give it to them. He has a hard time saying no to people. I sometimes don't know how we've kept the doors open. He saw a lot of people and didn't charge them. He's just that type of person."

Altruism has not affected Charles' business endeavors. He and

Calzada were able to invest in a new facility located in Germantown. A Panamanian ophthalmologist, Calzada had been mentored by the late Dr. Barrett Haik at the University of Tennessee early in his career and was becoming an accomplished vitreoretinal surgeon when he went on to be trained by Charles. For his part, Charles recognized the younger man's skills and business instincts and eventually offered him a full partnership in the retina institute. The choice was astute; Charles is disinclined toward the business details that Calzada knows are important to the future of their practice.

"This building, for instance, was my project," Calzada said. "I guess it was my pet project, and it was a big deal that he agreed to go along. Remember, biology doesn't allow us to live forever. Steve's doing his best, but nobody finally wins. I think he understood this building implies something of a legacy. And he recognized he needed to be involved. When we were doing the analysis, he said, 'You get the corner office, you pushed this forward, and you're going to be here longer.'

"I have very different ways of working," Calzada added. "I sweat the details, and he lets someone else do that. His objective self said, 'This building is the right decision.' His humble self probably found it uncomfortable when he walked in here."

Charles was, however, intimately involved in the new building and played a major role by doing the IT, VoIP, security, electrical, AV, HVAC, and exam room layout, and is responsible for half of the mortgage.

Calzada was talking to me from behind a broad desk in the corner office he had been promised. Charles' dozens of patents hung on the wall in a hallway outside the door, around the corner from Charles' own office. If Steve is as disengaged regarding business operations as Calzada suggests, his selection of a partner is another sound strategic choice. Calzada has always been protective of his partner's reputation and the legacy of the institute he built. He immediately understood what an honor it was to be invited into a partnership with Charles. Yet even with doctors committed to the generational torch being passed, the transition of certain responsibilities is not simple, emotionally or logistically. There are challenging practical matters to running a multimillion-dollar business.

"Do you think being married to him in the business world is easy?" Calzada asked. "It took a lot of effort. It matured me a lot because I had to manage my feelings. Steve knew he wanted someone strong next to him, but when you come down to nitty-gritty decisions and processes, it was very difficult for him to relinquish the amount of control necessary for me to get things done. I guess it was also tough for the people around him because some of them saw me as a threat to their environment."

Whatever sensitivities and apprehensions might have been perceived, they did not appear to cause major problems in professional or personal relationships at the Charles Retina Institute. When I toured the Germantown facility, I found myself thinking about Steve's whiskey-sipping paternal grandfather, a lumberjack who rode a railroad handcar to work in the northern woods of Wisconsin and became a surgeon who founded the Colon and Rectal Surgery Society. What would he make of his grandson's accomplishments in medicine, the list of patents, and his pioneering techniques and technologies? And surely Charles' mother's father would be impressed as well. An immigrant Swede and mechanical engineer who designed diesel engines and worked in the Elgin Watch factory, he gave Steve his interest in engineering, which led, ultimately, to the Constellation, the world's most sophisticated and successful retinal surgery platform.

The waiting room at the Germantown offices is always full.

Patients come from across the country and around the world to be treated here. At 75, Charles still sees 60-plus patients per day on Mondays and Wednesdays and operates on about 10 each Tuesday and Thursday. The indefatigable Sabrina Newsom continues to assist him, briefing the doctor on each case and making certain he accomplishes the day's tasks. The people who work with Charles have become a family, bound together by a common purpose around a central figure.

On one of my early visits to Memphis, I had been sitting in the dimly-lit waiting area of his old offices when my wife began a muted conversation with an older man waiting to see the doctor. She told him we were optimistic Charles might be able to restore my eyesight. The man, dressed in jeans and a work shirt, sighed and looked over at Mary Lou.

"Oh, he can," said the man, pleased with himself. "I wouldn't worry too much about it."

"My husband has already had a lot of operations and still can't see," she said.

"He'll be all right." The man paused. "You know what I call him?"

"Dr. Charles?" Mary Lou asked.

"I call him Doctor God. That's the truth. He seems like that to my family. He's fixed every problem my kids and I have ever had."

The three of us had no way of knowing he was talking to possibly the only family in that crowded waiting room—perhaps the solitary case Charles had encountered in years—that he could not help. Invoking a deity added another level or irony to the conversation. I am not given to religious inclinations or belief systems. In fact, I've found them to be absurd on various intellectual and cultural levels. As my friendship with Charles grew, I learned that he was respectful of the religious convictions of his patients, but his conversion, if it were ever to come, would be the product of science. He was driven by charitable impulses and a desire to help others, but his morality arose from personal kindness and required no religious dogma.

Alicia Joyner, a certified surgical and technical assistant at Charles Retina Institute who assists Charles in all surgical cases, met the doctor in 1983 when she was asked to substitute for an absent surgical technician.

"I guess I just started asking him questions," Joyner said. "And our first case was a detachment and then a diabetic retinopathy. I couldn't believe how great it was to restore someone's vision, how wonderful that felt. He said, 'Alicia, I want to see you in my office.' I went in there, and he said, 'I'd like you to come work with me. I am opening up my own practice.' I said, 'Yes, sir, I really appreciate the opportunity.' He told me that he was impressed I had shown interest and wanted to learn."

In the ensuing years, Charles has been Joyner's doctor, employer, and friend. He raced to the hospital when she was losing her father, and when her house tragically burned to the ground, she looked up to find Charles at her shoulder and ready to offer help.

When I finally got Charles to sit for a conversation in his office, the subject matter invariably turned to the state of the American health-care system. The doctor has long been frustrated by physicians' needs to worry about issues like coding, compliance, risk management, cost containment, and even billing. Details like these consume inordinate amounts of time and personnel and drive an inattention to providing up-to-date and the highest-quality patient care. He also thinks many doctors spend too much time on golf, collecting, and investments and not enough on continuing their medical educations.

"I'd be embarrassed to be seen on a golf course or in a movie theater," Charles said. "And art and wine talk bores me. I want to focus on important things. Look, we spent over $2 trillion in Iraq, and we're still spending. We killed one million noncombatants and probably didn't help anything. And Washington tells us we don't have enough money for NIH research, Medicare, Medicaid, or to properly fund even the Affordable Care Act? We've got a lot of things wrong."

In fact, Charles insisted he had not taken a vacation since 1996 and had not been to a movie in 30 years (except a few with his grandchildren) and has not played golf, gone fishing, or been to a wine tasting. He is constantly worried about the future of American health care and issues like the imbalance that is occurring between compassionate, informed patient care and a high-tech medical practice that requires imaging and electronic medical records (EMR). He believes something important is lost as doctors spend their time looking at computers, lab data, and EMR and hardly touch or even talk to their patients. The fact that 60 percent of U.S. physicians are employed by hospital systems also concerns him, since competing priorities like management and efficiency issues can, when not properly overseen, overemphasize revenue and constrain patient care.

There is, of course, no way to completely disentangle the delivery of health care in America from business, and revenue is one of the key measures to value an invention. What happened to MicroDexterity, one of Charles' start-ups, is a case in point. The effectiveness of his robotic designs in bone surgery led Stryker to invest in the firm and eventually to buy it for $50 million. Later, however, Stryker executives chose to compete in knee replacement instead of orthopedic bone surgery. As a result, MicroDexterity and its products ceased to exist, a decision driven, perhaps, by profits, not patients.

Stryker's failure to promote and market MicroDexterity's

robotics was frustrating, but Charles was not going to give up his technological ideas for "advanced visualization for spine, neurosurgery, and trans-oral approaches to head and neck cancer, and anterior skull base." That is, essentially, the mission statement for his latest technology business, CamPlex. Charles had been thinking for some time that surgical outcomes in these areas could be improved with better optics and a "heads-up" option for the physician.

"I had this idea way back when I was working on MicroDexterity's robots," Charles said. "I was having some anxiety and a bit of frustration about where things were going to go with that project, and I needed an outlet for my engineering skills. I began to think about putting really small cameras on the ends of surgical tools and retractors. It wouldn't be like an endoscope or a separate micro camera. This would be a completely new approach."

Charles intends to build tiny high-definition cameras that would be placed at the end of retractors and other surgical tools. The images would be fed back to a sterile touch screen that doctors could see in the operating room. The display would allow them to choose what they see through a binocular display unit, a microscopic viewer. The surgeons would always be able to see where their instruments are and how they are being used. And they could see it all in 4K definition. Charles' team is also designing the CamPlex system with "folded optics," which bends and focuses light while it is passed back and forth inside of an optical system. The clarity of the video will be unprecedented.

I heard the details of this latest idea in Charles' office during a break in his patient routine. When he stepped out to resume his consultations and exams, I found myself wondering how he would succeed with CamPlex, given his attitude toward conducting business. Inventions do not get to the marketplace without a business plan, investment, manufacturing, marketing, and distribution. Yet all those are things Charles has historically left to partners and hired professionals, which is probably why he has never been completely satisfied with the results. Unfortunately, these are also tasks he simply cannot devote himself to with the same fervor he applies to surgery and invention. Still, he keeps going.

A copy of Steve's book, *Vitreous Microsurgery*, was on a shelf in his office, and I opened it while I waited for him to return and resume our conversation. The fifth edition, including artwork by in-house graphic artist and photographer Byron Wood, has been translated into six languages. Wood's illustrations offer a clear understanding of the interior of the eye and what the instruments are doing, or need to do, during each procedure. I referred to the book countless times as I was trying to understand the biology of the eye, the complications I had endured, and the techniques Steve had created to fix problems like mine.

The book has prompted colleagues, patients, and friends to ask Charles why he never became a medical school educator. Clearly, he has the capabilities to teach in a major university, run a research lab, train residents, and give lectures. Most people think that is a natural habitat for someone of his intellect and energy. There has never been even the slightest hint, though, that Charles might be interested in the ivy-covered walls of academe. His teaching, in fact, already has a broad reach through the fellows at the Charles Retina Institute—some of whom have become leaders in the field—his lectures at teaching hospitals and clinics, observers who come to his clinic, and demonstration surgeries that are often widely broadcast via the Internet and closed-circuit TV or offered as training aboard the Orbis Flying Eye Hospital.

Charles is not cut out for academic gowns and research committees.

"Those guys work a few hours a day," said vitreoretinal surgeon Robert Laborde, a former Charles Retina Institute fellow. "They might also work a few more overseeing their labs. They lead a cushy life and publish a lot, and Steve just doesn't play those types of games. He wants to be a busy clinician, and he wants to operate and develop technology; Steve does not care about that tenured professor world. He doesn't want to wear a gown and be a distinguished prof at Duke. I think he could certainly be the chair of a department at Wills [the Philadelphia eye clinic], but Steve is just wound way too tight to go to those committee meetings and deal with the crap to be an academic professor. He will always be too driven to slow down."

Spending time in the clinic with patients, writing patents, performing surgeries, and designing sophisticated technology does not leave Charles an abundance of hours to write articles for peer review or constantly attend symposia. His legacy may be slightly diminished by his disinterest in publishing in medical and engineering journals, but he does not waste time contemplating his place in vitreoretinal history. He believes his contemporaries and those he has taught will ensure his legacy through the use of his ideas and inventions. He has always been at his best when he is doing things that solve problems.

Stephen Huddleston wanted to make certain I understood the breadth of what the doctor had accomplished. "Steve is definitely the greatest living advancer of retina," Huddleston said. "And he does get a lot of credit. But even so, he doesn't get credit for the big retina B-Scan he created, which makes no sense. And the hand piece he still has—it's used everywhere. Think about what a difference that's made! Back in the '80s, before that device, they'd take an eye out thinking it had cancer, and it was just blood. People used to go crazy taking eyes out for stuff, and docs thought they had something, but they often didn't. People are just dogmatic. But Steve's work has added information to prevent these things."

Charles is not without his critics, but writing about his life and work risks having the story viewed as a hagiography. Undoubtedly, some colleagues have found him off-putting. The doctor has never hesitated to share his opinions or research findings, and they often conflict with conventional practices.

As an example, Charles has not used a scleral buckle in retinal repair for almost two decades because he believes other approaches are less problematic for patients. Scleral buckles cause an average 2.75 diopter change to increase myopia, which, Charles has long argued, is unacceptable to patients who have paid for LASIK or have had lenses implanted to fix cataracts. Strabismus, or wandering eye, can also be a side effect, along with pain, incarceration of the retina, bleeding, and even perforation of the retina.

Charles is not a rebel by nature; he simply has no patience with diplomacy when it comes to advancing medicine. His friend Eric Donnenfeld, a world-class cataract and corneal surgeon, thinks that is a major benefit both to the profession and people struggling with retinal issues.

"Steve doesn't have what you might call a controller," Donnenfeld said. "He doesn't [hold with] political correctness, and he doesn't mind stepping on toes. Maybe a small part of his intellect enjoys being a renegade. But he does what needs to be done, regardless of what convention dictates. Convention is meaningless to him. He looks at a problem and says, 'Ignore everything done in the past.' He isn't burdened by previous information, and because of that, it changes what everyone else does in ophthalmology. Steve just moves forward right through what others can't seem to ignore."

Richard Lindstrom, a widely respected ophthalmologist, has

always believed that Steve was set apart from others simply by destiny, which is probably not the type of assertion one might expect from a man of science and medicine.

"I do think some of us are chosen to be special," Lindstrom told me. "And those that are chosen get to make special contributions. I expect that to some extent Steve was one of those people. When he was 22, I don't think he had it all mapped out. But I think Steve Charles was chosen. And God bless us for the fact he was who he was and recognized his obligations to his great mind and talents."

Certainly, Charles has managed to find ways to bring together his inventions and surgery and to combine them with his love of aviation. The Sabreliner he flies with Buddy Dawsey makes it possible for Charles to consult for Alcon in California and Texas, perform high volumes of surgery, and teach where he is called. But even helping a company produce sight-saving equipment can lead to criticism. A mild rebuke of his book in an Amazon review suggested that he mentioned Alcon too often in the manuscript. Yet Charles is a paid consultant to the company, and they used his architectural designs to build the Accurus and Constellation platforms, which have earned the company billions. Without that relationship, the technology might have developed anyway, but perhaps not as quickly. And who knows how many people might have lost their vision in the interim?

Charles makes no apologies for who he is and what he does.

"My prime interest is in giving care and fixing eyes," Charles told me that afternoon in Germantown. "I have a calling of advancing the craft and teaching those advancements to others, so it doesn't just help my patients but other patients anywhere my machines and techniques might be used. I make money on technology. And I feel like I continue to become more efficient and more organized.

I am at peak form now in terms of developing things and doing surgery. I wrote about 30 patent applications with Alcon in the last calendar year. And I confess I like this feeling of being well regarded on the podium."

After my interviews had concluded and I was heading south out of Memphis through the loblolly pine forests of Mississippi, I was once more wishing that I had met the doctor before the vision in my right eye was not recoverable. There was an inevitable sadness in my predicament, but I was adjusting to a monocular existence. And he had become a friend I expected to keep close for the rest of my life. On that sunlit southbound highway toward Texas, I decided that, regardless of the timing, I was fortunate to have met and become friends with Steve Charles, M.D.

SEVENTEEN

A Man without Repose

His rhythms hardly ever change. Monday mornings, he is up around 5:00 a.m. to begin exercise, weights, or cardio for more than an hour. Then, he drives to the Charles Retina Institute in Germantown. On an average day, Dr. Steve Charles will see 60 patients about problems with their vision caused by retinal issues. Many of them will be scheduled for surgery the next morning or on Thursday of the same week. He performs his operations Tuesdays and Thursdays at the Hamilton Eye Institute at the University of Tennessee Health Science Center in Memphis. On Fridays and weekends, Steve Charles often travels for product-development engineering to do teaching operations or to lecture.

At 75 years of age, the doctor shows no signs of decline or intentions to quit learning and providing care. Charles and his associates have taken out a 15-year mortgage to finance their new offices and clinic—not the sign of a man who is thinking about sleepy mornings and leisurely evenings on a tropical veranda.

"Steve is a very driven and positive person," said his friend and colleague George Williams, chair of ophthalmology at the William Beaumont School of Medicine at Oakland University. "This is a man who knows himself, and he's taken great care of himself. Steve is in superb physical condition and literally can run someone 20 years his junior into the ground. He works and studies as hard as he does without quitting, because he has come to the conclusion that 'This is who I am. This is what I do. And I enjoy it.' And he does. There really is no one like him."

No one perhaps knows the doctor better than his youngest daughter, Marci, who owns and operates Zip Lost Pines in Austin, Texas. Marci Charles does not completely buy into her father's obsessive profile and claims to have seen him ride a bike, watch a football game on TV, and water ski. Although her descriptions of her father in a state of relaxation have never been independently verified, she makes a compelling argument that the globally renowned surgeon-scientist-dad is driven, at least, in part, by fear of mortality.

"I've always sensed fear in him," she said. "He's been so worried about dying at a young age. He kept saying, 'I've gotta stay healthy. I've got things to do.' You can run yourself into the ground with anxiety about your health. He said, 'I don't want to die young. I've known too many people who've died young.' And then, I asked him if he was afraid of what's next. The look on his face was one of, 'What *is* next?' What if there is something, and you never thought there was? Doesn't that scare you? That's horrifying. I am certain my dad thinks about this a lot. He can't really envision what might come next because he is working so hard on what he's doing here and now. But maybe we all have to think about that."

Time may still make its ultimate claim on Charles, but there is no shortage of people who would be unsurprised if he also won that contest. He still does two or three more times the number of retinal surgeries in one day than most of the leaders in his field, many of the patients are sent to him because they are too challenging for other vitreoretinal doctors, and he continues to work with the engineering and development teams at Alcon for the next generation platform that will replace his Constellation vitreoretinal surgery platform. The doctor's determination and dedication are unflagging.

He has passed his work ethic on to his three daughters by maintaining persistent involvement in their lives through two failed marriages. Two of them are doctors and maintain busy practices. Kelli Charles Ross is a Florida gynecologist, and Kerri Charles has a family practice in Colorado.

"I remember him taking us around the hospital," Kerri Charles said, "and being at the clinic with him when we were kids. I loved being there watching him do his work, and I remember how much he loved it. I always hoped I loved my job that much. He has always been the guy who said you can do anything. He has never thought that anything isn't achievable, if you work hard enough. Growing up, it never occurred to me there isn't anything I couldn't do; I could be an astronaut or a surfer or Olympian, whatever I wanted. My dad gave me that."

Charles' level of performance may be exceptional, but he is not unique in his desire to stay on the job. According to the American Medical Association, 21 percent of the one million physicians in the United States are above the age of 65, and 42 percent are older than 55. The most important issue associated with aging for doctors, and especially surgeons, is staying current with new techniques and technology, which may be as demanding of a doctor's time as a heavy patient load. Orthopedic surgeon Ralph Blasier wrote in 2009, "Every treatment technique taught 25 years ago has been abandoned and replaced." In Charles' case, and in his area of specialization, keeping up with developments is usually simpler because he is often the leading innovator.

Still there is no escaping the degradation of human function caused by time. The clock breaks everyone. A surgeon in his seventh decade is arguably not the same talent that he was at 50, though he may be more skilled. Charles spent those two decades learning, designing new tools, improving surgical techniques, and finding ways to reduce risk and improve outcomes for his patients. The assumption some could make is that Charles ought to be confronting a moral quandary brought on by his age: When is the time to retire? Will he recognize when he is no longer as capable of performing microsurgeries inside of the eye?

Some of Charles' colleagues and friends may wonder whether the doctor would know if his time of repose had arrived. Fine motor skills always deteriorate. The moment will come, inevitably, when his hand is not steady, the eyes not as clear, and he will be the first to know and make the right decision. No one watching the doctor work now, however, can envision when he might quit. Such a day still seems incomprehensible to those closest to Charles.

Robert Laborde, a vitreoretinal surgeon and a former Charles Retina Institute fellow, noted there are no indications that his mentor and friend ought to stop helping people see.

"It's too late to worry about him," Laborde said. "I asked him once if he was going to retire. The question almost felt irrelevant. For some people there would be tremor in the hand. But I see a lot of older patients. Some people age hard, and some don't. Remember the effort Steve puts into taking care of himself. I don't see a moral quandary for him about when to retire. I know if he wasn't able to perform and operate at his level of expectations with the right outcomes that he would shift to teaching or something else. I think it's also important to understand that the wrist performs the most delicate parts of retinal surgery. You use a rest, and you use your fingertips. The retina is very unforgiving if you happen to screw up. But Steve has very high expectations and strong ethics about outcomes. He will never put anyone at risk."

There are, in professional, scientific, inventive, and creative endeavors, people who transform expectations and standards of excellence. Charles sustains that type of influence and relevance over vitreoretinal surgery more than five decades after he became a doctor. Many of his colleagues, in fact, believe most of the improvements being made in retina are simply fine tunings of advancements he first achieved. The essential steps to reattaching most retinas involve hydraulics like draining subretinal fluid while infusing air; they are not likely to be significantly altered.

There also seems to be a consensus among retinal specialists that the accelerated evolution of technology and techniques in their profession is a consequence of Charles' innovations. No one doubts his advancements might have transpired eventually, but virtually everyone acknowledges that retinal surgery took a leap forward in the wake of Robert Machemer's first vitrectomy—which looks almost crude today—because Charles was a determined surgeon with great engineering skills. His success in engineering, surgery, and teaching has given him a transcendent reputation.

"He's almost like a character in one of those Greek tragedies with their single-focused heroes," said Tarek Hassan, M.D., a past president of the American Society of Retina Specialists. "He's the most focused guy I have ever seen. And, yes, he's almost a mythic figure. There are just not people like that who have no hobbies, nothing else but what they do, and love it like he does; he's so wrapped up in the field."

Although Machemer's Vitreous Infusion Suction Cutter (VISC) opened the doors to surgeons in the retina subspecialty, Hassan thinks comparisons between the father of vitrectomy and Charles are not very compelling.

"I remember Machemer, and when he retired from Duke, the guy closed the door and never looked back, never went to meetings, no longer was involved in innovation. He was done and gone by choice. One day this great man, Robert Machemer, walked out the door, and they never saw him again at the OR or on the podium. To this day, Steve is relevant, active, and engaged, way more than other people in our profession. Steve is always trying to better his mind. But I sort of worry about the guy sometimes."

Talking only about Charles' skills as a technician underemphasizes his personal connections to patients and his reputation as a man who has never said no to friends in need. The number of people who want to see the doctor can also leave the wrong impression he is more clinical than caring. He learns as much as he can about his patients' conditions, not their vacations, new cars, or their children. He does, however, have a facility for connecting with the people he treats.

Sabrina Newsom is Charles' closest medical assistant. She moves through the halls of the Charles Retina Institute in front of the doctor, making certain patients are ready when he walks in for their examinations, digital images are on screens, and patient files are available. The adroit ministrations of Newsom and her colleagues are part of the reason Charles is able to see so many people. But Newsom thinks it's a mistake to consider Charles too clinical and businesslike.

"I know that I am working for a doctor who really cares about his patients," she said. "I've been here for a long time, and I've never seen him go at anything other than 110 percent. I think that's just bred into him. He wouldn't be happy any other way, and he's been like that, I'm sure, for every day he's practiced. People learn very quickly that he's one of the kindest, most caring people they can meet. He's never turned anyone away. When patients say they don't have insurance or money for a needed operation, he tells them not to worry about it, that he'll pay for it. We are all proud to work for Dr. Charles."

The professional associations of retinal specialists continually note the doctor's achievements. As Charles was beginning to plan his trip to China with the Orbis Flying Eye Hospital, he was asked to make a stop in San Diego. He was about to receive one of the greatest honors in his long and storied career.

THE OCULARIST WHO designed and painted the pupil of my prosthetic eye covering had given me a short rubber stub with a concave tip. By wetting the end and pressing it against the hardened acrylic scleral shell, I created hydraulic suction that allowed me to pull it out of my eye socket. I do this every few months for cleaning, and at that time I am confronted with what remains of my natural eye. Shriveled and crossed by veins, the surviving globe has the appearance and bumpy surface of a poorly boiled egg left in the sun to dry. An accumulation of mucus almost always sits on the surface near the dark spot that used to be my pupil but now looks like a festering bruise.

My inclination is to always avoid looking at the dead eye when I clean the prosthesis. No one, I suspect, wants to confront one's physical frailties. I have avoided letting my wife or daughter see what has happened to my eye. I have told them what it looks like, but they do not know what to say and tend to look at me as though I have just described an alien visitor from a distant galaxy.

I suspect the prosthesis, as natural as it appears, probably cost me a very nice consulting contract. The presentation I gave to a technology start-up was very strong. I provided executives with a lucrative go-to-market strategy, and a logical and achievable plan to add strategic partnerships. The company was bound to grow, and my advice should have given them confidence in their future and in me.

But I never heard from them again.

Winning business is always far from certain, but I can usually sense when I have been persuasive. However, when I stopped by the restroom on the way back to my truck, I realized I was probably not going to get the work. In the mirror I saw that the prosthesis had slipped to one side; my eye appeared to be looking off to the side of my head. I was horrified. No wonder the company's CEO had been giving me an oddly quizzical stare. I thought, mistakenly, his reaction was about how I had come up with such brilliant business plans. My instinct was to center the prosthesis and go back up for some trivial reason and let them see me looking normal, but I chose to simply go home.

The stability of the prosthesis is not a significant problem. However, there are times when it is dry, and if I blink hard, my eyelids will grab at the surface and move it. And if I reach up to scratch near the eye or rub it, that, too, can push the prosthesis out of position without my awareness. People will look at me strangely until I realize I need to find a mirror.

My solution was to start carrying a pocket mirror, the type that often comes with expensive contact-lens-solution kits. If I sense that my prosthesis has slipped from its centered position, I quickly pull out the mirror and take a look. I have become quite skilled at holding it beneath a table and glancing down while I am in meetings or at restaurants with clients or friends. Only on one occasion, during a holiday barbecue at a friend's home, was I caught with the mirror and asked to explain.

"What the hell?" a buddy asked. "You fixing your makeup?"

"No, I've got something in my eye."

"And you happen to have a mirror in your pocket?"

"Yeah, happens a lot with these contact lenses."

There has never been a rational reason for not telling my friends about the loss of my eye. A few are aware, because they knew what I was enduring through years of operations. My openness is restrained, I have decided, in much the same psychological fashion as people who are given a dire diagnosis of cancer. Many of them never tell a soul outside of their families and closest friends because they refuse to be defined by a disease. They don't want to be transformed from writer, ballerina, ballplayer, politician, or surgeon into a person who is dying of cancer and fighting a "courageous battle" against a horrible disease. None of us wants to be considered victims of circumstance. We want to decide who we are and how we are perceived by the world. I am not, therefore, a monocular man to anyone but my family and a few friends (though I suppose this book will change that).

Outside of financial challenges caused by losing business and money and living on credit cards through my surgeries, I am unchanged. I still take pleasure in riding a big motorcycle through the Texas Hill Country or the Trans-Pecos, hiking in the Chisos of Big Bend or any of the other national parks, and spending hours in the saddle of my road bicycle, pushing my heart to levels that approach what they were when I was a young marathoner and steeplechaser. I read most books on tablets that allow me to adjust text size in order to minimize the stress on my single eye. I write white papers, books and blogs, and commission opinion pieces for CNN, and I continue to consult for start-up technology businesses in Austin. I work hard and take nothing for granted.

I do not, however, play baseball any longer, though I think about the game frequently enough to make myself melancholy on occasion. Watching professional players does not assuage my longing. The sport is connected to my youth, and, as a few American poets have suggested, to a yearly rebirth of possibilities we know exist but cannot name. Such expressions are artless overreaches for me. I always loved the simple fact that each pitch presented the chance to be a hero with a diving catch or a critical hit, a stolen base or a perfect throw to nail an overly optimistic base runner. Even into my early 60s, before I lost my eye, I was able to exercise those skills with a degree of proficiency.

The risk of playing now, though, is too great. My good eye would face the pitcher, and a hit to the temporal region might cause retinal detachment. There is also the chance that I might dislodge my remaining healthy retina by sliding into a base or diving for a ball. I realize I take chances riding my motorcycle and bicycle. But those are not prohibitive risks. The odds are far less that I will get into an accident and harm my eye than if I am facing 30 baseballs thrown my way during the course of a game.

I have to settle for memories of the game and watching others play, and I am adjusting to that notion. To have chased a spinning baseball across the green outfield carpet and made an improbable catch is a joyful remembrance. And nothing can ever erase what it felt like to stroke a three-run homer over the center-field fence to give my team the victory when there were two outs and two men on in the bottom of the ninth. On hot days, when I played first base, I loved to pick up handfuls of dirt and feel its warmth in my hands, then hold the glove to my face and smell the leather and sweat, and experience all the emotions of those sensory triggers.

It is, perhaps, just another silly sport, but its angles and outcomes and images and smells feel as though they comprise muscular memory and tissue striations in my body. Some part of baseball will always make up the essence of my character. I will permanently be emotionally attached to ballparks and their promise and the sound of a bat on a ball, to the absurd athletics of talented players, and the vague assurances of life's continuity that the game offers each spring. Though I can no longer play, I continue to experience the beauties of baseball.

And I can still see.

IF THEY WERE expecting great introspection and deep emotional revelations, they had chosen the wrong man to honor. Steve Charles is not the type to look back unless the memory informs what he wants to see transpire in front of him. He had been named to receive the Retina Research Foundation Award of Merit at the annual meeting of the Retina Society in San Diego, California, in September 2016. As the honoree, Charles was expected to deliver the Charles L. Schepens Lecture, which he entitled, "Evolution of Vitreoretinal Techniques and Technologies."

The event was an august gathering of great physicians and thinkers, at least one of whom was a decent comedian. Dr. Kirk Packo was asked by Charles to provide an introduction. After listing the doctor's major achievements, Packo offered what he considered the full roster of the surgeon's inventions. These included, but were not limited to, tequila, the iPad, the pressure cooker, yellow highlighter pens, nose-hair clippers, polio vaccine, the printing press, the cotton gin, the helicopter, the ballpoint pen, the Slinky, and dozens of other creations that seemed only slightly satirical to people who knew Charles and his capabilities.

Packo then showed a slide of Charles with a tube coming out of the rear of his surgical scrubs and plugged into a vitrectomy machine and suggested the doctor had invented "The First Flatulence-Powered Vitrectomy Cutter." His funniest take on Charles, however, had to be his description of a typical day in the life of history's most driven vitreoretinal surgeon:

5:00 a.m.	Works out lifting weights and 5K run
6:05 a.m.	Breakfast: bowl of kale
6:15 a.m.	Eight conference calls & 350 emails
7:00 a.m.	Baptist Hospital OR Room 6—performs 184 vitrectomies
12:00 p.m.	Lunch: tofu slices and carrot juice
12:15 p.m.	Meditation to extend his telomeres
1:00 p.m.	Office patients—sees 422 post-ops
4:30 p.m.	12 conference calls & 425 emails
5:05 p.m.	Edits the 23rd edition of his book
6:00 p.m.	Dinner: fried chicken and grits
6:15 p.m.	Skypes with daughters and grandchildren
8:00 p.m.	Invents something
8:05 p.m.	Invents another thing—patents both inventions
8:15 p.m.	Changes his mind—invents something else
8:30 p.m.	Reads 30 engineering journals, 10 robotics texts
10:00 p.m.	Works out again
11:00 p.m.	Practices on jet simulator in his basement
12:00 a.m.	Dresses up in an Elvis impersonator's jumpsuit and dances
1:00 a.m.	15 conference calls & 627 emails
2:00 a.m.	Edits the 24th edition of his book
3:00 a.m.	Learns to speak Sanskrit

3:30 a.m. *(Unknown . . . Drapes were drawn . . .)*

4:00 a.m. Sleeps

By the time Charles had finished his lecture after the comic introduction, his professional colleagues might have been convinced that Packo's daily log was not wildly inaccurate. The title slide, "Techniques and Technologies Evolve in Parallel," teed up a historical analysis of the advancements of vitreoretinal surgery. Many of the important milestones had his name attached. These included cutting action and the design and improvement of vitreous cutters, aspiration fluidics, and the aggregation of tools and techniques into surgical platforms like the Ocutome 8000 and Alcon's Constellation.

He also reported on the fluid, air, and gas exchange and one of the most important markers in vitreoretinal achievement—internal drainage of subretinal fluid. There was also a list of tactics he employed in the switch from a single port to three-port vitrectomy, the ideas he developed for approaching proliferative vitreo retinopathy (PVR) surgeries, retinopexy with lasers, the advantage of re-operations without removing previously injected silicone oil, and what he described as a "two-port 25-gauge silicone oil re-op" methodology.

Although he certainly had to feel pride at being recognized for his unprecedented achievements, Charles was not emotional. This was a man doing what he has always done with great capability: teaching, explaining, sharing, motivating, and inspiring by actions rather than words. Afterward, Charles came as close as he probably ever does to considering the end of something great. A number of his friends approached him with handshakes and hugs, including Dr. George Williams from Michigan, who suggested Charles begin contemplating his personal legacy.

"He asked me if I thought about it," Charles said, "and where I planned to donate money. He said, 'When you have it, why don't you donate $250,000 to the academy for a Steve Charles lecture? There's a Schepens Lecture; there needs to be one with your name on it. You've developed all of the stuff we use worldwide.' And I said I will do that."

Charles had already donated his $40,000 honorarium for the Schepens Lecture back to the Retina Society to further its educational efforts. As he chatted with well-wishers, he had to keep explaining that work was his form of celebration and that his three daughters were not in attendance because they had jobs and lives and commitments.

Charles was not bothered by their absence. Although he liked being honored and appreciated for his achievements, the doctor has never been the type to get choked up or gush about how wonderful it was to be feted or flattered.

"I was hugely honored, of course," he said. "But instead of motivating me to chill and be celebratory with friends, I just felt it made the point that I needed to roll up my sleeves and get back to work. It's nice to be told you did a good job. But I work because I work—that's the best explanation. I love retina and engineering and learning and teaching. My reaction to getting this honor was that not too long afterward I went to my hotel room, managed some emails, and wrote two patent applications for Alcon."

The San Diego awards ceremony and lecture were simply a stop on the road to a different place and another task. Charles was en route to China as part of the first mission of the MD-10 version of the Orbis Flying Eye Hospital. After the flight from Los Angeles to Shenyang, Charles was to spend his first day, a Sunday, delivering a symposium on "Surgical Retina," which would be followed by the screening of 26 or 28 patients at the He University Eye Hospital. He was scheduled to perform 10 surgeries on the giant jet.

Before leaving to catch his long trans-Pacific flight to China, Charles turned slightly introspective.

"I guess it's a different way of thinking about things," he said, "but I recently considered the fact that I am probably flying my last airplane. I'll never buy another one. I'm living in my last apartment; I've got my last truck. I guess I've also gotten used to living alone and being alone, and being devoted to my work. I expect to operate for another decade or two. That's why I maintain discipline of exercise and diet. I want to keep doing this."

Paul Runge, M.D., who had been a fellow at the Charles Retina Institute and took his medical degree from the Flinders University of South Australia School of Medicine, has been a friend of Charles for almost four decades and cannot envision the doctor's decline. "I bet," Runge said, "if we have this conversation in 10 years, he will be doing exactly what he's doing now and will have new innovations. I think he has much better balance in his life now than even 10 years ago. I am pleased that he is still working and helping so many people, including practicing physicians like myself. We constantly try to keep up with his new innovations. If anything, the world needs more like Steve Charles, not less. We are all so fortunate to have him helping us improve the care we give the eye and helping people to see."

When he finally climbed steps up to the giant Orbis MD-10 parked at the airport in Shenyang, Charles undoubtedly stuck his head into the flight deck. He cannot resist being around airplane technology and controls. He always wants to say hello and talk to the people who fly aircraft, understand their systems, and share his love of aviation. Charles probably also noticed the plaque that had been attached to the back of the co-pilot's seat. The text memorialized Charles' $100,000 donation to Orbis in honor of the friends who had been driving forces behind the dream of an airborne hospital.

It read, "Steve Charles, vitreoretinal surgeon, engineer, and jet pilot, donated this seat to honor Al Ueltschi, Oliver Foot, Jack McHale, FedEx, and Alcon."

Charles did not linger long on the flight deck. He was scheduled for multiple teaching surgeries that day. He hurried to the operating room at the back of the airplane. The Constellation surgical platform was secured against the wall, ready to be deployed in retinal repair. Steve said hello to his colleagues, asked questions about the patient's prep, and moved into the operating theater without further distraction.

The doctor was ready to get to work.

A Note about Sources

The primary source for this narrative was, of course, Dr. Steve Charles. He sat for long interviews in Austin and Memphis and was constantly available via phone, text, and email to answer my ongoing questions, which were, seemingly endless. To get an understanding of medical procedures on the eye, I also relied greatly on his book, *Vitreous Microsurgery* (Lippincott, Williams & Wilkins, 2011, fifth edition), which included the gloriously detailed imagery by Charles Retina's staff artist, Byron Wood. The book was published in multiple languages and was co-authored by Steve's business partner, Jorge Calzada, M.D. The text and accompanying visuals made it possible for a layperson to understand the structure of the eye and how surgery manipulated tissue to save vision.

My debt is also great to the medical masterwork entitled, *Vitreous: in Health and Disease* (Springer, 2014), J. Sebag, M.D., editor. Any question on the intraocular space and biology of the eye, surgical advancements and understanding of vision, can seemingly be answered by the numerous professionals who contributed to the lengthy text. The writing and detail were certainly intended for the physician, but it is accessible to those without professional training. I found the work invaluable to enhancing my understanding of the exquisite beauty of anatomy that is manifested by the function of the human eye.

The other sources cited in this book are the numerous physicians, researchers, engineers, inventors, and patients that are all quoted in the text. There are only two quotes taken from the public domain;

I did not interview Napoleone Ferrara, the Genentech researcher who created the drug Avastin, which has all but ended wet macular degeneration caused by diabetes. I would certainly hope to speak with him someday, and I personally expect that he will, eventually, be awarded a Nobel for Medicine.

I read an uncounted number of medical tracts and articles regarding developments in ocular surgery and drug advancements. If they were of note or value to my narrative, they were used and cited. My goal was to write an authoritative story of a great man and avoid burdening the text with footnotes and dozens of pages of back matter added to the book. My part of the story, in which I describe my struggle, is, obviously, derived from my experience as a patient of nine retinal surgeries. The details of those operations were drawn from my doctor's post- operative notes, which he gave to me before I had decided to write a book but when I was deep into trying to understand what had happened to me.

I had no intention of writing a textbook. My goal was more biography and narrative. I did want to educate the reader about the life and accomplishments of Steve Charles, but I did not want to leave them with the impression that they were about to slog through a medical publication like a post-grad student heading for their M.D. The goal was an approach that let the reader know the information I was conveying was authoritative and came from peer-reviewed articles, expert interviews, and sources that have been verified as accurate and true. My interest was not in slowing down an engaging story with an overabundance of footnotes. I wanted people to hear about Steve Charles and learn of his achievements.

I believe this methodology has worked, and *Give Back the Light* will provide a record of this exemplary man's life. I had no other ambition with this project.

Acknowledgments

Books originate in less than mysterious ways. An author might overhear a conversation that triggers an idea, or a life's work could lead to a summation in narrative form. An original and inspiring story can be lying about and stumbled upon by an enterprising dreamer. Inspiration is hard to define but has to be mixed with determination to create a manuscript.

This book began over tacos. In fact, the concept emerged over barbacoa tacos (flour tortillas, always) at Maria's in South Austin during a conversation with my friend Robert Bryce, the prolific author of books about energy and the initial critical analysis of the Enron collapse, *Pipe Dreams.* Robert and I had not seen each other in a few years, and I began to tell him about the problems with my eye. The story of dealing with the health care system and meeting Steve Charles as I struggled to save my vision intrigued Bryce, who immediately urged me to turn it into a book.

"It's a hell of a narrative," I recall him telling me, "and you've got this amazing person in the middle of it. Not you, of course."

"Okay, wiseass. I hear you. But I am just through with several years of dealing with this, and I am not sure I want to relive it."

"I can understand," he said. "But doesn't change the fact that it's an interesting topic, and you are a writer."

I spent the next few months trying to avoid the subject of Dr. Charles and my eye problems, but there was no question Robert was right, and I had just been through a pivotal moment in my life with a person of some historical importance. But I was also busy with my business consulting practice, and science and medicine could hardly be considered my areas of expertise. Nonetheless, the idea persisted, and I began the process of educating myself on biology, medicine, and engineering, and later began a draft that I doubted would ever make sense or have any appeal. Disciplined as I was, I had great skepticism I'd ever see the book to its end.

Two years and seven months later, I had a manuscript.

I am grateful to Robert Bryce for providing the idea for *Give Back the Light.* There are, of course, dozens of others who have facilitated the completion of this publication, either directly or indirectly. My greatest debt, obviously, is to Steve Charles, M.D., whose days of healing and learning are far too busy to afford a writer any of his time. The doctor, however, was gracious and endlessly supportive, not just helpful. I hope this book serves to offer an additional legacy for his great accomplishments in the field of vitreoretinal surgery and the difference he has made in the lives of uncountable people. Honoring his life and work were my primary motivation.

There is an extensive list of ophthalmologists that also indulged me for interviews. Many of them are quoted in the text, but they all contributed greatly to my understanding of the beauty and precision of their profession and the endeavor of saving eyesight. These physicians include Juan Amaral, M.D., who is leading a stem cell project on dry macular degeneration; Kirk Packo M.D., a raconteur, brilliant surgeon, and unofficial historian of ophthalmological surgery; Carl Regillo, M.D.; Chris Blodi, M.D.; Don D'Amico, M.D.; Eric Donnenfeld, M.D.; Emmett Cunningham, Jr., M.D.; J. Fernando Arevalo Colina, M.D.; George Williams, M.D.; the late Barrett Haik, M.D. of the University of Tennessee's Hamilton Eye Institute, where Steve performs his surgeries; Joe Robertson, M.D.;

Dr. Charles' business partner, Jorge Calzada, M.D.; Julia Haller, M.D.; Steve's daughter, Kerri Charles, M.D.; Richard Lindstrom, M.D.; Richard J. Mackool, M.D.; Robert Laborde, M.D.; Andy Packer, M.D.; Mohammad Rafieetary, O.D., F.A.A.O.; Robert Spetzler, M.D., the neurosurgeon who operated on Steve's carotid occlusion and was his neurosurgical consultant in MicroDexterity robotics; Paul Runge, M.D.; and Dr. Charles' newest practice partner, Stephen Huddleston, M.D. The artwork of Byron Wood, whose illustrations are published in Dr. Charles' book *Vitreous Microsurgery,* were instrumental in educating me on the basics of the eye and how treatments of the retina were accomplished in surgery.

My limited understanding of mechanical and electrical engineering was greatly enhanced by Bruno Dacquay; Carter Cliff; Jean- Marie Parel, Ph.D., one of the many foundational geniuses of Bascom Palmer Eye Institute; and Ken Charhut, Michael Papac, the late Michael Stuart, and Paul Hallen, who all spent time working with Dr. Charles on various projects as he developed technology for Alcon and his personal startup businesses involving robotics, surgical platforms, tools, and optics. Their insights were invaluable to the author. Jack McHale, an aircraft expert and buyer for FedEx, helped me with the history of the Orbis Flying Eye Hospital and the genesis of its great philanthropic work, which came about also because of McHale's energy and commitment.

Any success I have on this book, like the daily achievements of Dr. Charles, is connected to his diligent, enthused, and intelligent staff at the Charles Retina Institute in the Memphis suburb of Germantown. I began with the indefatigable Sabrina Newsom, who seems to manage every detail regarding patients and Charles' day and is constantly striding in front of him when she is not at his side. I also want to thank his surgical assistant, Alicia Joyner;

Jeanne Linville for scheduling assistance and regular updates; and Judy Perry, who manages the doctor's finances, all of whom made this project much more enjoyable and informed.

I got a greater insight into Steve Charles as a person through family and friends of the doctor, including his daughters, Marci Charles and Kerri Charles, M.D., who, unsurprisingly, think their dad was as good at being a father as he is at being a surgeon. Daughter Kelli Charles Ross, like her father, also became a talented surgeon and practices gynecology and obstetrics. Steve's longtime co-pilot of his Sabreliner jet and the other aircraft he has flown through the years, Buddy Dawsey, who may know Steve as well as anyone given the time they have spent together in travel, taught me pointers on aviation and why Steve is also an exceptional pilot and an even better friend. Dawsey, like the man he flies with, is one of the best at his profession and was honored by the F.A.A. with a 50-year recognition of achievement. He can fly anything with wings.

I am also greatly indebted to a few of Steve's patients. Carl Daniel shared with me the great fear he experienced when his teenaged son began to lose his sight and told me how Dr. Charles' skills and financial generosity saved the boy's vision. Mark Mullen, whose courage defies understanding for me, told of transitioning his life to complete darkness and how Steve gave him years of light before helping him as a child and a man to accept that his biology could not be overcome. And Judge Kevin Norwood explained how the doctor who repaired his eyesight when others could not became a friend of profound importance in his life.

Thanks also to Gerald Helzner, a journalist who specializes in writing about the human eye and, in particular, the retina. He offered his experience and perspective on the development of pharmacological and technological approaches for dealing with retinal problems, which he developed after decades of writing for top medical publications.

The final stretch of this book was drafted in idyllic surroundings on the shores of Lake Huron up in Michigan, thanks to the generosity of wonderful friends Helen Curran and Cleosia Seay. They provided their cottage as a place of quietude and focus, and I was never more productive than during that month near the big water.

The only reason I have any type of accomplishment in my life is because of my wife and daughter. Even as a young woman, Amanda Noelle still thinks her dad is magical and can do anything, but whatever ends up on my ledger that is good and valuable has much to do with my bride, Mary Lou Pagels Moore, the little red-haired girl from Bro-Fen Farm in Birch Run Michigan; her faith has never faltered.

James C. Moore
Austin, Texas

The Major Honors and Lectureships of Steve Charles, M.D.

Vitreous Society (now American Society of Retinal Specialists): First Founders Medal

Club Jules Gonin: Herman Wacker Prize

Retina Society: Charles L. Schepens Lecture

American Society of Cataract and Refractive Surgery: Kelman Lecture

University of Miami Leonard Miller Medical School: Alumni Hall of Fame

Ridley Medal

American Academy of Ophthalmology: Laureate Honoree (October 2018)

Hawaiian Eye & Retina Corboy Award (2019)

The Patents of Steve Charles, M.D.

Title	Current Status	Application, Publication, Grant Number	Inventors
One Handed Syringe	Granted	3,993,064	Charles, Steven T. (EXT_STC)
Chin Activated Switch	Granted	4,045,630	Charles, Steven T. (EXT_STC)
Linear Intra-ocular Suction Device	Granted	4,395,258	Charles, Steven T. (EXT_STC)
Method of Performing Ophthalmic Surgery Utilizing a Linear Intra-Ocular Suction Device	Granted	4,493,698	Charles, Steven T. (EXT_STC)
Vitreous Cutter	Granted	5,176,628	Charles, Steven T. (EXT_STC)
Tubing Management System	Granted	5,464,025	Charles, Steven T. (EXT_STC)
Decoupled Six Degree of Freedom Robot Manipulator	Granted	5,710,870	Charles, Steven T. (EXT_STC)
Decoupled Six Degree of Freedom Teleoperated Robot System	Granted	5,784,542	Charles, Steven T. (EXT_STC)
In Vivo Polymerizable Ophthalmic Compositions	Granted	5,858,345	Charles, Steven T. (EXT_STC)
Master-Slave Micromanipulator Apparatus	Granted	5,943,914	Charles, Steven T. (EXT_STC)
Master-Slave Micromanipulator Method	Granted	6,000,297	Charles, Steven T. (EXT_STC)
Coordinated X-Y Stage Apparatus	Granted	6,016,607	Charles, Steven T. (EXT_STC)
Articles Coated With In Vivo Polymerizable Ophthalmic Compositions	Granted	6,124,037	Charles, Steven T. (EXT_STC)
In Vivo Polymerizable Ophthalmic Compositions and Methods of Using	Granted	6,180,687	Charles, Steven T. (EXT_STC)
Parallel Mechanism	Granted	6,330,837	Charles, Steven T. (EXT_STC)

Continued

Gradient index surgical illuminator	Granted	7,824,089	Charles, Steven T. (EXT_STC)
Spiral Scanner with Electronic Control	Granted	6,626,834	Charles, Steven T. (EXT_STC)
Medical Manipulator for use with an Imaging Device	Granted	6,665,554	Charles, Steven T. (EXT_STC)
Surgical Manipulator	Granted	6,676,669	Charles, Steven T. (EXT_STC)
Vitreoretinal Instrument	Granted	7,141,048	Charles, Steven T. (EXT_STC)
Vitreoretinal Instrument	Granted	7,285,107	Charles, Steven T. (EXT_STC)
Ergonomic Footswitch	Granted	7,193,169	Charles, Steven T. (EXT_STC)
System for actuation of a vitreous cutter	Granted	8,080,029	Charles, Steven T. (EXT_STC)
Viscous fluid extraction	Granted	8,251,980	Charles, Steven T. (EXT_STC)
Variable drive vitrectomy cutter	Granted	8,298,253	Charles, Steven T. (EXT_STC)
Devices, systems, and methods for pupil expansion	Granted	8,852,091	Charles, Steven T. (EXT_STC)
Interface for viewing cameras on a surgical visualization system	Granted	8,882,662	Charles, Steven T. (EXT_STC)
Infusion pressure control using blood pressure	Granted	8,658,948	Charles, Steven T. (EXT_STC)
Gradient index surgical illuminator	Granted	7,824,089	Charles, Steven T. (EXT_STC)
Docking station with temperature control and electronic identification system	Granted	8,905,930	Charles, Steven T. (EXT_STC)
Devices, systems, and methods for pupil expansion	Granted	8,852,091	Charles, Steven T. (EXT_STC)
Handle for ophthalmic surgical instrument	Granted	D612052	Charles, Steven T. (EXT_STC)
Ocular Unit for Eye Surgery (OCM)	Granted	D325, 086	Charles, Steven T. (EXT_STC)
Systems And Methods For Reinjection Of Processed Vitreous Humor	Granted	9549849	Charles, Steven T. (EXT_STC)
Infusion Pressure Control Using Blood Pressure	Granted	9415162	Charles, Steven T. (EXT_STC)

Method And System To Detect Ophthalmic Tissue Structure And Pathologies	Allowed	2014-0307078	Papac, Michael J. (papacmi1); Yadlowsky, Michael J. (EXT_MY); Charles, Steven T. (EXT_STC)
Infusion Pressure Control Using Blood Pressure	Granted	8905930	Charles, Steven T. (EXT_STC)
Gradient Index Surgical Illuminator	Granted	7824089	Charles, Steven T. (EXT_STC)
Docking Station With Temperature Control And Electronic Identification System	Granted	8658948	Charles, Steven T. (EXT_STC)
Ergonomic Footswitch	Granted	7193169	Charles, Steven T. (EXT_STC); Mezhinsky, Victor B. (CPI17392)
Viscous Fluid Extraction	Granted	8251980	Zica, Michael Arthur (CPI17762); Bazydlo, Matthew Edward (CPI23930); Charles, Steven T. (EXT_STC)
Variable Drive Vitrectomy Cutter	Granted	8298253	Charles, Steven T. (EXT_STC)
System And Method For Actuation Of A Vitreous Cutter	Granted	8080029	Charles, Steven T. (EXT_STC)
Vitreoretinal Instrument	Granted	7141048	Charles, Steven T. (EXT_STC)
Vitreoretinal Instrument	Granted	7285107	Charles, Steven T. (EXT_STC)
Devices, Systems And Methods For Pupil Expansion	Granted	8852091	Sussman, Glenn Robert (sussmgl2 (external)); Charles, Steven T. (EXT_STC); Chin, Hsin Sheila (CHINS)
System And Method For Identifying And Controlling Ophthalmic Surgical Devices And Components	Granted	7934648	Malk, Edward (CPI17332); Charles, Steven T. (EXT_STC)
Devices And Methods For Active Head Stabilization During Surgery	Publication of Application	2016-0175178	Charles, Steven T. (EXT_STC)
Ophthalmic Surgical System With Blue Light Filtering	Granted	9386918	Ammari, Eyad (EXT_EA); Charles, Steven T. (EXT_STC)
Infusion Pressure Control Using Blood Pressure	Publication of Application	2014-0276558	Charles, Steven T. (EXT_STC)
Infusion Pressure Control Using Blood Pressure	Granted	9655776	Charles, Steven T. (EXT_STC)

Continued

Variable Stiffness Cannula And Methods For A Surgical System	Granted	9730834	Charles, Steven T. (EXT_STC)
Increased Depth Of Field Microscope And Associated Devices, Systems, And Methods	Granted	9844314	Charles, Steven T. (EXT_STC); Papac, Michael J. (papacmi1)
Extended Depth Of Focus Contact Lens For Vitreoretinal Surgery	Publication of Application	2017-0188825	Charles, Steven T. (EXT_STC); Smith, Ronald T. (Theodore) (smithrok)
Vitreoretinal Instruments For Fluid Aspiration Background	Filed	62/485154	Grueebler, Reto (gruebre1); Schaller, Philipp (schalph1); Charles, Steven T. (EXT_STC)
Active Noise Cancellation In An Ophthalmic Surgical System	Publication of Application	2018-0018953	Todd, Kirk Wellington (EXT_TKW); Ekvall, Johan Gustaf (EXT_EJG); Essex, Paul J. (essexpa1); Charles, Steven T. (EXT_STC); Gunn, Nicholas Max (EXT_NMG)
Resolution Enhancement Of Oct Images During Vitreoretinal Surgery	Publication of Application	2017-0228858	Charles, Steven T. (EXT_STC)
Oct-Enabled Injection For Vitreoretinal Surgery	Filed	62/572599	Charles, Steven T. (EXT_STC)
Foot Pedal Controlled Oct-Display For Vitreoretinal Surgery	Filed	62/577773	Charles, Steven T. (EXT_STC); Heeren, Tammo (EXT_TH1)
Membrane Delamination Device	Publication of Application	2017-0360603	Grueebler, Reto (gruebre1); Linsi, Thomas (linsith2); Wolfer, Rodolfo (wolfero2); Vigaru, Bogdan (vigarbo1); Charles, Steven T. (EXT_STC)
Subtractive En Face Optical Coherence Tomography Imaging	Filed	15/695608	Charles, Steven T. (EXT_STC); Yu, Lingfeng (YULIF); Ren, Hugang (EXT_RH1)
Stereo-Optic Surgical Contact Lens	Publication of Application	2017-0105620	Charles, Steven T. (EXT_STC)
Contact Lens Mounting Speculum For Vitreoretinal Surgery	Granted	9877648	Farley, Mark Harrison (FARLEMA1); Charles, Steven T. (EXT_STC)
Ophthalmic Surgical System With Blue Light Filtering	Granted	9849029	Ammari, Eyad (EXT_EA); Charles, Steven T. (EXT_STC)
Subretinal Fluid Drainage Instruments, Systems, And Methods	Publication of Application	2018-0042768	Charles, Steven T. (EXT_STC)

Surgical Apparatus Including Aspiration Device Sensors	Publication of Application	2018-0049920	Charles, Steven T. (EXT_STC)
Binocular En Face Optical Coherence Tomography Imaging	Publication of Application	2017-0135573	Charles, Steven T. (EXT_STC)
Membrane Delamination Devices	Filed	62/472337	Grueebler, Reto (gruebre1); Linsi, Thomas (linsith2); Wolfer, Rodolfo (wolfero2); Vigaru, Bogdan (vigarbo1); Charles, Steven T. (EXT_STC)
Cannula With Optical Sensing	Publication of Application	2017-0172667	Charles, Steven T. (EXT_STC)
Mechanical Attachment Between Surgical Microscope And Indirect Contact Lens	Grant	9854969	Smith, Ronald T. (Theodore) (smithrok); Heeren, Tammo (EXT_TH1); Charles, Steven T. (EXT_STC)
Methods And System For Imaging An Inner Limiting Membrane Using A Stain	Publication of Application	2017-0245754	Charles, Steven T. (EXT_STC)
Ophthalmic Illumination System With Light Intensity Control On Individual Illumination Fibers	Publication of Application	2016-0346058	Hallen, Paul R. (hallepa6); Charles, Steven T. (EXT_STC); Smith, Ronald T. (Theodore) (smithrok); Bacher, Gerald David (bachege2); Ammari, Eyad (EXT_EA); Papac, Michael J. (papacmi1)
Fogging Prevention For Surgical Contact Lenses	Publication of Application	2017-0319062	Charles, Steven T. (EXT_STC)
Surgical Probe With An Integrated Motion Sensor	Publication of Application	2018-0055592	Heeren, Tammo (EXT_TH1); Charles, Steven T. (EXT_STC)
Devices And Systems For Stabilization Of Surgeon's Arm During Surgery	Publication of Application	2017-0172698	Charles, Steven T. (EXT_STC)
Vital Stain Visualization In Ophthalmic Surgical Procedures And Associated Devices, Systems, And Methods	Publication of Application	2016-0270649	Papac, Michael J. (papacmi1); Charles, Steven T. (EXT_STC)
Automatic Lens To Cornea Standoff Control For Non-Contact Visualization	Filed	62/508617	Charles, Steven T. (EXT_STC)

Continued

Vitrectomy Probe With Rotary Cutter And Associated Devices, Systems, And Methods	Publication of Application	2018-0008463	Charles, Steven T. (EXT_STC)
Systems And Methods For Pulsed Posterior Vitreous Detachment Creation	Publication of Application	2016-0346122	Charles, Steven T. (EXT_STC)
Curvature Of Field Transformation Of Oct Images During Vitreoretinal Surgery	Publication of Application	2017-0135574	Charles, Steven T. (EXT_STC)
Resolution Enhancement Of Oct Images During Vitreoretinal Surgery	Granted	9649021	Charles, Steven T. (EXT_STC)
Ophthalmic Visualization Devices, Systems, And Methods	Granted	9693686	Smith, Ronald T. (Theodore) (smithrok); Yu, Lingfeng (YULIF); Papac, Michael J. (papacmi1); Olivera, Argelio Michael (EXT_AMO); Charles, Steven T. (EXT_STC)
Systems And Methods For Pressure-Driven Tool Actuation	Filed	15/862192	Charles, Steven T. (EXT_STC)
Mechanical Support Of An Indirect Contact Lens By A Surgical Microscope During A Vitreoretinal Surgery	Filed	15/846464	Smith, Ronald T. (Theodore) (smithrok); Heeren, Tammo (EXT_TH1); Charles, Steven T. (EXT_STC)
Automatic Lens To Cornea Standoff Control For Non-Contact Visualization	Filing decision		Charles, Steven T. (EXT_STC)
Ophthalmic Surgery Foot Pedal Device Having Force Feedback	Filing decision		Charles, Steven T. (EXT_STC); Sorensen, Gary P. (sorenga1)
Contact Lens Mounting Speculum For Vitreoretinal Surgery	Filed	15/875178	Farley, Mark Harrison (FARLEMA1); Charles, Steven T. (EXT_STC)
Foot Pedal With Force Feedback	Filing decision		Charles, Steven T. (EXT_STC); Sorensen, Gary P. (sorenga1)
Vitreoretinal Instruments For Fluid Aspiration	Filing decision		Grueebler, Reto (gruebre1); Schaller, Philipp (schalph1); Charles, Steven T. (EXT_STC)
Surgical Instrument Using Detected Light	Filed	62/633866	Charles, Steven T. (EXT_STC)

Vacuum Control For A Vitrectomy Probe	Filed	15/866828	Charles, Steven T. (EXT_STC); McDonell, Brian William (mcdonbr4)
Surgical Retractor	Granted	9,492,065 13/802,362	Charles, Steven T. (EXT_STC)
Surgical Visualization System With Camera Tracking	Granted	9,615,728 13/802,162	Charles, Steven T. (EXT_STC)
Hydraulic System For Surgical Applications	Granted	13/802,635	Charles, Steven T. (EXT_STC)
Interface For Viewing Video From Cameras On A Surgical	Granted	8,882,662 13/802,509	Charles, Steven T. (EXT_STC)
Interface For Viewing Video From Cameras On A Surgical Visualization System	Granted	9,681,796 14/537,524	Charles, Steven T. (EXT_STC)
Binocular Viewing Assembly For A Surgical Visualization System	Granted	9,629,523 13/802,582	Charles, Steven T. (EXT_STC)
Surgical Visualization System	Granted	9,642,606 14/215,826	Charles, Steven T. (EXT_STC)

About the Author

James C. Moore is the *New York Times* best-selling author of *Bush's Brain*, the first critical examination of the George W. Bush administration, and five other books of fiction and nonfiction. He is an Emmy-winning former TV news correspondent, an on-air TV political analyst, op-ed writer for CNN, and a technology startup business consultant. Mr. Moore has traveled extensively on every presidential campaign of the last forty years and has written and reported on most of the major historical news events of that era. He lives in the Central Texas Hill Country outside of Austin with his wife and daughter.